POST-MORTEM

POST-MORTEM

David M. Spain, M.D.
with Janet Kole

Doubleday & Company, Inc.   Garden City, New York

ISBN: 0-385-01905-X
Library of Congress Catalogue Card Number 73–83674
Copyright © 1974 by David M. Spain
All Rights Reserved
Printed in the United States of America
First Edition

CONTENTS

III. MADISON AVENUE MURDERS

PREFACE

The decision to write this book stemmed from something said to me by Dick Gregory, the humorist and civil-rights activist. He may have been joking, but I took him seriously. In any case, immediately upon my return from Mississippi (where I had gone at the behest of the families to investigate the deaths of the three young civil-rights workers who had been kidnaped, murdered, and dumped into a clay pit), Dick Gregory, David Welch of *Ramparts* magazine, and I appeared on Long John Nebel's radio show. After the show, the three of us went out for a drink and Gregory told me that he had warned his wife to contact me immediately in the event of his death. He was convinced that he was marked for assassination by white racists and wanted to be sure that I would perform the autopsy so that the truth about how he died would not be hidden. His request actually anticipated an entirely new area of pathology in which I soon was to be involved, and which in the next few years occupied a good measure of my efforts, thoughts, and time.

"Civil-rights pathology" added a vital dimension to my career, which until then had consisted of teaching, research, hospital pathology, and medical-legal work. It supplemented the bizarre and often sensational aspects of human behavior I had encountered in my previous years as a pathologist, when, especially as a medical examiner, my daily environment had been saturated with cases of murder, suicide, violent accidents, criminal abortions, and infanticide.

Some of the crucial components of this story have to do with the physical autopsies on the victims, but an equally important part comes out of conferences with the relatives or friends of the deceased, and official dialogue with lawyers, reporters, influence peddlers, investigators, police, undertakers, psychopaths, and crackpots. These daily events made me a witness to, and frequently a participant in, many startling "moments of truth." I had the opportunity not only to examine the dead hearts dissected at autopsy, but also the live hearts of those caught in the webs of these deaths. Death was the final event for the victims; for them it was all over. But from these fatalities were generated the courtroom scenes, the murder trials, the criminal investigations, the contested wills, the personal recriminations, and the feelings of guilt these chapters discuss.

My medical-examiner days were over long ago, but my advice and counsel in related matters are still sought by troubled families, attorneys, and, on rare occasions, by government agencies. My experience as a pathologist was enriched by tours of service with the National Study Group on Smoking and Health, with a research study group of the American Heart Association, and by continuing research into various aspects of sudden death from "heart attacks."

Actually this book explores, through the major cases of unnatural death in which I have been involved, the uses of the autopsy as a truth-seeking tool of medicine and the law. Every chapter centers around at least one real-life case. All are concerned with the basic question of civil rights and liberties—that is, the protection of the individual from a vested interest,

whether that vested interest be the government accusing someone of murder or a tobacco company selling cigarettes.

All of these cases have represented for me a continuing struggle against bias and prejudice (prejudice being an emotional
response to the threatening of one's vested interest). Although
there have never been any total victories in this search after
truth, each partial victory makes the truth a little easier to find
than it was before.

It would seem that unremitting exposure to so much ugliness,
pain, and deceit would instill a cynical and despairing view of
humanity. However, the contrary is true: the endless numbers
of meaningless and needless deaths were constant and potent
reminders to me of the precarious and delicate balance in which
each solitary, frail, and sacred human life is sustained. I re-
sisted the potentially dehumanizing effect of years spent with
the lifeless at the dissecting table and amid shelves lined with
jars containing cut-up bits of former life, by a self-imposed
daily routine of silent prayer composed of the words spoken
by Shakespeare's Hamlet: "What a piece of work is a man!
how noble in reason! how infinite in faculty! in form and moving
how express and admirable! in action how like an angel! in
apprehension how like a god! the beauty of the world! the para-
gon of animals!"

It might seem from my portrayal of events that I have remarkable inductive powers. This is decidedly not the case. A
pathologist examines the facts, after the event is over. He is
dealing with hindsight—like the person who says, "I told you
so," or the proverbial Monday-morning quarterback. The
pathologist's not-so-secret intellectual tool, the "retrospecto-
scope," creates this illusion of exceptional personal insight.

Many years have elapsed since the occurrence of most of
the recorded happenings. To prevent any personal embarrassment, harmful exposure, or unintentional misrepresentation of

persons still alive or the awakening of painful memories, I have
altered or deleted names, places, and time where necessary.
In no instance have the essential facts of any event been
changed.

There was truth and there was untruth, and if you clung to the truth even against the whole world, you were not mad.

George Orwell

The place where men come together to seek the truth is holy ground. The autopsy room is such a place.

I

POLITICS CAN PLAY HAVOC
WITH THE FACTS

1. RACISM IN WESTCHESTER

That justice is a blind goddess
Is a thing to which we black are wise.
Her bandage hides two festering sores
That once perhaps were eyes.

Langston Hughes

I had always intended to become a general practitioner. To train myself thoroughly and sharpen my diagnostic ability, I decided to spend a year as a resident physician in the pathology laboratory at Kings County Hospital, in New York City. During that year, I became deeply intrigued with pathology, the specialty that studies changes in the tissues of the body caused by disease or injury and is usually practiced in a hospital lab. But at the end of the year I was still intent on becoming a family doctor.

My intentions were undermined when I suddenly became ill with a serious kidney infection. Upon recovery, I was told to take it easy for a while and work regular hours. So, until I was back to health, I decided to continue to work as a pathologist. Thirty years later, I'm still at it.

My reaction to my first autopsy was one of intense intellectual curiosity. The only time I became faint was the first time I saw a surgeon cut boldly into the tissues of a live body. My emotional reaction to dead bodies has varied with my knowledge of each individual case and the circumstances of the death. To this day, for example, I am still upset at the sight of a dead child, and must force myself to perform the necessary duties.

By the 1940s, modern medical technology and scientific knowledge, as we know them, were just coming of age. So was forensic pathology. Through the use of X rays, photographs, refined ballistics tests, dental identification, high-powered microscopes, and tissue slides, we were finding out that dead men do tell tales. (Now, with more advanced technology, they tell longer ones.) I was fascinated by what could be learned from the dead and how this knowledge could be put to use.

When I was hired by Westchester County, in February 1949, I was charged with the task of revamping the outmoded coroner's office and replacing it with a modern medical examiner's office. A coroner, under the old system, didn't have to be a pathologist—or even a physician. He might be the town undertaker, or even a garage owner. Few autopsies were performed; those that were done were usually done by untrained persons. The coroner's determination of cause of death was usually no more than a guess. The coroner could also become involved in legal matters. He was empowered to hold court in the form of an inquest and subpoena witnesses to testify under oath. But he did not need to have any legal training. In short, he was neither fish nor fowl: he was not sufficiently competent in either the legal or the medical aspects of the problems to arrive at a just and intelligent verdict. (Unfortunately, there are still some of these old-style coroners around. They are rapidly being replaced by modern medical examiners.)

The medical examiner must not only be a pathologist but must have had training in the forensic (legal) sciences. His position is a non-political one and he attends exclusively to the medical aspects of the investigation. His main tools are the autopsy and the toxicology laboratory. He holds no inquests, subpoenas no witnesses. Those aspects are left to the jurisdiction and competence of the district attorney's office, to whom the medical examiner submits his medical report if indicated or requested.

It wasn't until I acted as medical examiner in the Mikulicz case that one of the decisive paths of my career finally began to take shape. Looking back, I believe that this was the most crucial of my early experiences as medical examiner. It was the forerunner by more than a decade of my intense involvement with the nationally prominent civil-rights cases of the sixties and seventies—the slayings of the three civil-rights workers in Mississippi, the murderous raid on the Chicago Black Panthers, the New Haven Black Panther trial, and the prison fatalities in the New York Tombs and Attica.

One of the first steps I took as the new medical examiner of Westchester County was to establish a service to transport to the central morgue those bodies that were to be autopsied. We hired Jim Florence as the department chauffeur and part-time morgue technician. He was to be my touchstone during the Mikulicz case*; I needed one, because at that time my naïveté about race hatred was extreme. I had even been surprised when I was house hunting in Westchester to discover that I couldn't live in certain parts of the county because of a "gentleman's agreement" not to sell to Jews.

I think Jim Florence first realized I needed educating when, at the beginning of our relationship, I sent him on an assignment to White Plains to pick up a two-month-old male infant unexpectedly found dead in his crib. An hour and a half after

* The case is a real one, but names, dates, and sequence have been changed to spare the participants embarrassment.

he left, Jim still hadn't returned. I was concerned and telephoned to Captain De Lee of the White Plains police. He was just going to call me, he said. "The family of the dead baby refused to release the body to Jim."

"Why?"

"Because they won't trust the body to a nigger. And I'm inclined to agree with them."

Under these circumstances, the medical examiner's authority overrides that of the police, and I ordered Captain De Lee to enforce the decision that the body be turned over to Jim. Jim never had any more trouble on that score.

I was indignant about the attitude of the family and Captain De Lee. Jim, however, had taken the whole affair with unruffled resignation. He was used to this kind of thing happening: he had lived most of his life in Georgia, and his outlook had been conditioned by his long experience in the South.

Nevertheless, I thought Jim's disillusionment was overdeveloped. At that time I believed that despite occasional unpleasant instances of racism, Northern justice was reasonably evenhanded. It was not until the Mikulicz murder trial that I experienced firsthand how the Northern judicial system operated when a white man killed a black.

It began on June 17, 1950, when I was called in to examine two bodies, still warm, lying on a street in Yonkers, victims of a street-corner shooting. I found two black men, both dead, each with a bullet in his body. We brought them to the morgue for autopsy. As in every case my office dealt with, I obtained statements from witnesses, as well as reports from police and detectives at the scene, from the deputy commissioner of public safety of Yonkers, and from our own investigator, all of whom had questioned the surviving brother of the two dead men and the owner of the bar where the crime had been committed.

We reconstructed the events leading to the crime as follows:

Joe Mikulicz, a former member of one of the many local police forces in the county, had visited several bars on the day of the killings, having a few beers at each one. His final stop was at a bar where the two victims and their brother had been chatting. Mikulicz knew the bartender, and when he saw the three black brothers, Mikulicz indignantly asked him in Polish: "How come you serve colored people?"

"I serve whoever has the money to pay," said the bartender, also in Polish.

"Well, make sure you wash my glass carefully," said Mikulicz.

"I wash all my glasses carefully."

The three Negroes finished their beer, walked out, and stood talking nearby on the street. Mikulicz hastily gulped the remainder of his beer and rushed out to the three men, pulled out his revolver, and shouted: "You don't think I'll kill you niggers, do you?" And then he fired two shots in rapid succession, striking two of the brothers. He pulled the trigger a third time, but the gun jammed and he threw it down. The third brother sped from the scene and ran for medical help. Mikulicz made his way home.

Within a few minutes, the police arrived to find the men lying dead. The bartender identified the assailant, and two detectives hastened to his apartment. Their arrival coincided with that of the Yonkers deputy commissioner of public safety. Mikulicz was sitting on his bed busily loading another gun and screamed out: "I just shot two niggers and I'm going back to kill that other one." According to the detectives and the deputy commissioner, Mikulicz was excited and flushed but revealed no outward evidence of having been physically assaulted. He made no mention of having been attacked. The detectives disarmed and arrested him. According to statements by Mikulicz and the surviving brother, neither the three men nor Mikulicz knew or had ever seen each other before.

The slain men were brought from the site of the crime directly to the autopsy room, which was now a scene of considerable activity. An identification technician was fingerprinting the two dead men. A police photographer had set up his lights and tripod and was photographing the bullet wounds from every angle. Portable radiology equipment was being positioned to X-ray the bodies to locate the precise points where the bullets were embedded in the bodies.

I had carefully reviewed the witnesses' evidence and the police reports, all of which were recorded on an official form of the county medical examiner's office. (This form is prepared in advance of the autopsy and enables the medical examiner to approach the autopsy with intelligence.) I put on my dissecting-room clothes, rubber apron and gloves, and measured the exact location of the entrance bullet wounds, which were in almost identical positions in the two bodies. In the meantime, a detective had arrived and informed me that the slain men were "clean": they had no known police records of any civil disturbance or criminal activity. Both had been regularly employed, were married, and had children. Their good records seemed to exclude the possibility that some jurors might partially justify these murders on the grounds of previous criminal activity.

In all bullet-wound cases, the questions I am expected to answer for the law-enforcement agencies, and eventually in court, are these: Could the wounds have been inflicted with the suspected murder weapon? At what range was the weapon fired? From what direction? And finally, though not relevant in this case, could the wounds have been self-inflicted, due to accident or suicide?

The answers to the first three questions depend on the character of the wounds; the answer to the last question becomes evident with the resolution of the first three. A wound can be self-inflicted only from a range within the subject's reach (except when some string or cord is rigged up to pull the trigger, in which case the contraption is usually found). Entrance wounds are generally divided into three types, depending on the distance of the weapon at the time of discharge. There are "contact," "arm's reach," and "distance" wounds. An entrance wound is usually smaller than an exit wound (when an exit wound is present). A "contact" wound is invariably split, scorched, with singed hair, and sometimes slightly blackened. The tissues beneath the skin are bruised. These features are present up to a distance of two or three inches with a small weapon and up to five or six inches with a larger weapon. An "arm's reach" wound (from about six inches to within two or three feet) reveals a split entrance hole and scattered tattooing produced by powder markings. Anything over two or three feet is regarded as a "distance" wound. The characteristics are the same if the shooting has taken place from sixty feet for a pistol and two hundred feet for a rifle. The wound, in this instance, is not split or tattooed but is soiled by the spin of the bullet, which wipes off its grime as it pierces the skin. In the Mikulicz case, the entry wounds were only soiled, indicating that the shooting had occurred from a distance of over three feet.

The course of the projectile is determined by tracing a line (as long as it continues on a straight course) beginning at the entry wound and running into the body along the track of damage produced by the missile. If the bullet strikes bone, it is usually deflected and its course suffers a significant and sometimes bizarre change in direction. In Mikulicz's victims, the bullets entered their abdominal walls and proceeded in downward directions at a 45-degree angle on straight courses piercing both men's aortas (the largest artery in the body), causing the brothers to bleed to death within minutes. The spent bullets were embedded in the spinal column.

These facts, plus the knowledge of the distance of the entry wounds from the ground with the men in an erect position, made it possible to calculate the level and direction and approximate distance from which the shots had been fired.

A portion of brain tissue and some blood were saved for analysis of alcohol content. Results of the test indicated only a minimal trace of alcohol and suggested that, in all likelihood, each man had consumed no more than one glass of beer. This quantity was too slight to have made them belligerent or to have altered their behavior. No abrasions or bruises or other wounds were found on their hands or elsewhere, and there was nothing else to imply that they had been involved in any physical altercation. The remainder of the examination revealed no further evidence of injury or disease. The bullets were removed from the spine, marked with the victims' initials, and turned over to the ballistics experts. For this we received a signed receipt.

Joe Mikulicz was booked on suspicion of homicide and held for possible indictment on a second-degree manslaughter charge; a county-wide protest meeting held at the Center, in White Plains, demanded that Mikulicz be charged with murder in the first degree. When the time came, Mikulicz was indicted and the grand jury did hand down a first-degree charge.

The next month, I was summoned to testify in court. By now, the case had gained the full attention of the country's Negro press, which discussed and speculated on the eventual outcome of this trial.

John Marbach, the assistant district attorney assigned to the prosecution of the case, was competent and well prepared for the trial. On direct examination by Mr. Marbach, I testified as to the cause of death; the distance and direction from which

the shots came; the identification of the bullets, which were
shown to have come from the weapon fired by Mikulicz and
later discarded by him at the scene; the insignificant amount
of alcohol found in the brain tissue of the victims; and the absence of any other bruises or marks that might indicate involvement in a fight. On cross-examination, the defense attorney
repeatedly and vigorously tried to challenge the validity of the
alcohol determinations in an attempt to show the slain men
were drunk and obstreperous. He also tried to shake my interpretation of the downward path of the bullets. I was convinced
that he had failed to persuade the jury that my findings were
inaccurate; I didn't see how anyone could doubt the thorough
and official report of the county laboratories, and the defense
attorney offered no meaningful scientific objections to it.

The witnesses for the state were impressive and highly respected, and included police officers, detectives, the deputy
commissioner of public safety, the bartender, the surviving
brother, friends, relatives, and employers of the victims, former
employers of the defendant, the ballistics expert, and the chief
medical examiner of the county (me). Their composite testimony tended to show the good character of the slain men; that
they had not provoked or attacked Mikulicz; that they must
have been shot by someone in a standing position from a distance of at least three feet; that the defendant was known to
have hostility for blacks; that he owned the murder weapon;
that he was seen in the act of shooting; that he had been drink-
ing beer all afternoon; that he had resented the presence of
Negroes in the bar; that he was seen loading another gun; that
he was known to be a man possessed of violent temper; that
he was an outstanding marksman, well versed in the use of a
variety of guns, and that the shooting could not have been
accidental.

A picture had emerged of Mikulicz as a man who for years

had harbored a deep and overpowering hatred of Negroes, who had a volatile temper, and who had a previous record of many acts of violence.

Finally, on a Friday afternoon, at 4:15 P.M., the assistant district attorney of Westchester County rose and said, "Your honor, the state rests." Thus ended a meticulous, logical, and detailed presentation of evidence by twenty witnesses which had taken ten full working days of the trial.

The defense began the presentation of its case, and I went back to my office and my research on heart attacks, lung cancer, and doctor-induced diseases. I did, however, follow the trial in the local newspapers and was flabbergasted when I read that Mikulicz had taken the stand in his own defense. He claimed that as he left the bar, he had been attacked by the two men, was knocked down, and while lying on the ground had shot them in self-defense. It was, therefore, no surprise to me when I received a call from Marbach requesting that I submit evidence for a rebuttal of this new story.

The next morning, I prepared two life-sized sketches of the slain men to illustrate the site of the entry wounds, the angle at which the bullets entered the body, the courses of the bullets, and the places where they were embedded. As I was finishing these diagrams, Jim Florence came in. Noticing the charts, he said: "Dr. Spain, I know you mean well, but you're wasting your time. Facts don't count. That white man—nothing is going to happen to him. Nobody cares about killing colored people." I agreed that Mikulicz would not pay the full penalty, but it was impossible that he could get off scot free. I told this to Jim. He didn't say anything, but he didn't have to. His expression of absolute disbelief was sufficient. The outcome of this trial was going to teach one of us a lesson.

A few hours later I was back in court, again as a witness for the state. The carefully drawn diagrams were placed in care of the assistant district attorney, who at the appropriate time would introduce them as evidence. My stay on the witness stand was brief and proved to be the most futile and frustrating minutes I ever spent in court.

The assistant district attorney began by asking if I had prepared charts to demonstrate autopsy observations showing the trajectory of the bullets. Before I could answer, the defense attorney rose to his feet and objected to the question. Without a second's hesitation, the judge sustained the objection. Then followed a series of questions that, to the best of my recollection, went like this:

ASSISTANT DA: Dr. Spain—when you autopsied the two slain men, did you note the location of the entry wounds and the course the bullets took in the bodies?

DEFENSE ATTORNEY: Objection, your honor.

JUDGE: Objection sustained.

At this point, the assistant district attorney paced back and forth, thought awhile, and looked at some notes.

ASSISTANT DA: Dr. Spain—at what height from the ground and at what angle did the bullets enter the bodies?

DEFENSE ATTORNEY: Objection, your honor.

JUDGE: Objection sustained.

ASSISTANT DA: According to your autopsy findings, was it possible for these men to have sustained the bullet wounds you described from a pistol shot by someone lying or sitting on the ground?

DEFENSE ATTORNEY: Objection, your honor.

JUDGE: Objection sustained.

The judge then motioned for the assistant district attorney and the defense counsel to approach the bench. In a voice inaudible to the jury, the judge said that this was improper testimony to be introduced in rebuttal, since this subject had already been covered in the original presentation of the state's case and

this material was only a more detailed elaboration of the previously presented facts. He said that at this time he would allow
only the introduction of entirely new evidence.

He may have been technically correct, but now that I've had
extensive experience in court, I realize that most judges would
have permitted this line of questioning in order to be certain
that the jury had a precise and vivid picture of these previously
presented facts. Because of the judge's rigid position, the assistant district attorney now realized that it was hopeless to
continue along this line of inquiry.

"No further questions," he said.

Whereupon I was dismissed as a witness.

The assistant district attorney did not think that the failure
to introduce the charts could materially alter the outcome of
the case, since all the pertinent information had already been
introduced in the original testimony. These facts clearly destroyed Mikulicz's contention that he had shot the men from
a prone position after having been knocked down by them. It
was impossible for the bullets to have entered the bodies while
traveling in an upward direction.

The case for the defense was brief. The lawyers made their
summations and the judge made his charge to the jury. He instructed the jury that who had fired the fatal shots was not in
question. This had been established beyond any reasonable
doubt to have been Mikulicz. The only issue, he said, was
whether Mikulicz was in danger or believed he was in danger
and for this reason acted in self-defense. To highlight this point,
the judge stated that if a man is approached by a stranger and
senses a threatening gesture—be it real or imagined—he is justified in acting in his own defense. What the judge did not say,
but what I believe may have been in everyone's mind, was:
especially if the stranger happens to be black.

Despite what I felt to be the judge's clear bias, the case

seemed cut and dried; and it surprised no one when the jury completed their deliberations in less than one hour. Only in retrospect did this haste appear obscene. Because, when the foreman of the jury stood up, he pronounced Joseph Mikulicz *not guilty*. Mikulicz was once again a free man, innocent in the eyes of the law of any wrongdoing. The slaying of two men—who happened to be black—was now proclaimed just by the due process of law practiced in a society of free and fair men.

My dismay at this contempt for the value of black lives was profound. I dreaded meeting Jim—my personal feeling of guilt as a white man made me ashamed. But Jim seemed unruffled. He had predicted—and expected—this conclusion by the jury. He had understood better than I had, because he had faced what all black people face every day of their lives, not only in the South but in urbane, sophisticated Westchester County, the home of foundation presidents, university professors, educators, lawyers, doctors, diplomats—a county with no tradition of lynchings, church burnings, or race riots. Joe Mikulicz shot those men years before civil rights for blacks became a national issue, before white backlash became a fashionable northern pastime, and before fear of personal violence stalked the streets of cities and suburbs. Thus had justice been dispensed.

Twenty years of experience have tempered and modified my original harsh judgments of the jury, judge, and defendant for the verdict of not guilty. In addition, my concepts of justice and punishment have broadened and mellowed a bit beyond the simplistic "good guy versus bad guy" view I held as a fledgling medical examiner. Particularly grievous and dangerous at that time was my intense emotional involvement and concern with the outcome of the case. This was and is inexcusable in a medical examiner. The occupant and his office must always remain a neutral and objective seeker of the facts, and his observations must be interpreted and presented dispassionately.

Too often have some medical examiners behaved as if they were in and of themselves the judge, jury, and prosecutor. Ever since the Mikulicz case, I have repeatedly subjected myself to a merciless self-scrutiny to avoid repetition of this pitfall. The arrogance of inexperience and of ignorance had led me to assume that the official weight of my office should have been more than sufficient for the jury to unhesitatingly accept almost anything I had to say. Looking back, I certainly had no right to assume this and should have anticipated the strategy of the defense and been prepared with diagrams of the bullet paths at my initial court appearance. This would have solidified my testimony and obviated the later, unsuccessful attempt to present this additional information in court. What I was lacking then was humility.

At the time of the trial, I was almost totally unable to grasp any of the deeper emotional and symbolic features of the case —the motives that not only moved the judge and jury but also might have triggered the defendant to kill at the moment he did. Certainly Mikulicz was not just an aberration and a psychopath, but was more typical than I realized—differing mainly in that he was slightly ahead of his time. The jury certainly was not one amorphous mass of bigotry. I am convinced now that they were essentially decent people, honestly believing that they had acted fair-mindedly; they were totally without knowledge or perception of the slow, continuous, and corroding influence of prejudice over the years. As for the truth of Jim Florence's feelings, these would have been crystal clear if at the time I had had sufficient insight to heed the full significance of another Yonkers episode, which preceded the Mikulicz case by several months.

One night about 1:00 A.M., I was summoned to a bar located in a predominantly black area of Yonkers. A young white police officer had just shot and killed a Negro who had allegedly gone berserk from too much whiskey and "was tearing the place apart." The officer, in response to a call, had entered the bar and was immediately attacked by the wild drunk, who came at him with a broken beer bottle. In self-defense, the police officer fired at the man, who died almost instantly. Before leaving my home, I requested police headquarters in Yonkers to ask the undertaker closest to the scene to send a hearse and stand by to pick up the deceased. This was our usual practice, because the department's transport service was available only during the day. The police sergeant at the desk urged me to hurry, since news of the killing had spread through the entire neighborhood, and already many people were gathering and milling around in the street with increasing tension. When I arrived in Yonkers, a police escort was needed to get me through the now angry crowd. Once in the bar, I learned that a cordon of blacks had formed around the area and had stopped the undertaker's hearse, driven by a white. A spokesman for the people in the street kept shouting that no white undertaker would be permitted to remove the body. Accordingly I at once arranged for the only nearby black funeral director to come to the scene. Meanwhile the crowd was becoming more restless. Fortunately a hearse driven by a Negro arrived in time to abort a riot. After inspecting the bullet wound and ascertaining the surrounding circumstances, I sent out word to assure the mass of people that there would be a fair investigation. Only then was the black undertaker allowed to remove the dead man.

Most of the blacks in the street that night could not accept that the shooting might have been justified; even the few who conceded that the officer had no choice but to shoot in self-defense argued that he didn't have to "shoot to kill." This incident grew out of the kind of feeling Jim Florence had tried to convey to me during the Mikulicz case: the black man is not going to get justice at the hands of the white man. When the blacks near the tavern refused to release the dead Negro's body to a white undertaker, they were trying to change that fact by taking an action to safeguard their rights. A thorough, and I believe fair, investigation of the circumstances surrounding the shooting that night did take place. The officer was exonerated of any wrongdoing, and the unhappy black community seemed to accept the verdict as just. At least they made no visible sign of disbelief. Nevertheless that incident twenty years ago was, in embryo, the expression of what we now call Black Power. If I had had the insight then that I have now, it might have been possible for me to appreciate what Jim Florence was telling me.

2. MISSISSIPPI AUTOPSY—GOODMAN, SCHWERNER, AND CHANEY

Make them live in a valley of fear . . . a valley guarded by our men, who will be both their only hope and the source of their fear.

Adolf Hitler, 1939

My younger son, Robby, like most kids of his age, is concerned about the spreading violence and potential for ecological disaster we are faced with today, and wonders if he will be able to do anything about these things as he grows into a career. He asked me recently if I had any idea, when I chose it, that pathology would be a politically useful profession. The answer is no, I never did.

I first began to realize pathology's potential in a general way following the Mikulicz case, when it became obvious that the everyday problems I faced—lung-cancer deaths caused by cigarette smoking, deaths related to drunken driving, deaths from furtive illegal abortions—could be alleviated only through public education and legislative reform. I, more than most, was in a position to tell people what I knew was wrong and how it could be stopped.

Unfortunately, not all pathologists are willing to realize their responsibilities in this area. It was not until my involvement in the case of the three civil-rights workers who were murdered in Philadelphia, Mississippi, in 1964 that I began my participation in the civil-rights struggle.

Many people have wondered what a New York pathologist's link was with a Mississippi murder case. My link was Arthur Kinoy, who is now considered one of the country's leading experts in Constitutional law. I had had no previous acquaintance with him until a less publicized civil-rights case brought us together professionally.

In that case, a sixteen-year-old black youth had been convicted and sentenced to death, in Alabama, for the alleged rape of a white woman. He was tried before an all-white jury and had only a perfunctory defense, by court-assigned counsel. This summary dispensation of justice, along with the excessively harsh sentence, gained the attention of some civil-rights groups. Arthur Kinoy entered the case and won from Supreme Court Justice Douglas a last-minute stay of execution. Under Kinoy's guidance the case was fought through, and the Supreme Court rendered a landmark decision ordering a retrial because the youth, Seal, had not been judged by a jury of his peers: the panel from which the jury had been selected contained no blacks. Also, the court found that Seal had not had access to an adequate defense.

Kinoy asked me if I would review a transcript of the medical testimony from the original rape trial and then prepare a medical rebuttal for the retrial. I had no difficulty doing what he asked. This is the ridiculously poor quality of the medical testimony contained in the transcript, as the prosecuting attorney, Mr. Booth, questioned Dr. Frank Johnston, who had examined the rape victim.

A. "She had—on a smear in spite of the amount of water and a bit of oozing blood from the cervix, the opening into her womb, she had live spermatozoa, which I carried the specimen myself to the laboratory. I checked it in the presence of one of the nurses."

Q. "Was that live spermatozoa male, or not?"

A. "That is what male sperm is, spermatozoa."

Then the court-appointed defense attorney, Mr. Johnson, questioned the doctor.

Q. "Doctor Johnston, you do not know how she came to be in that condition, do you?"

A. "I do not know how she came to be in this condition. I saw the patient lying on the table."

Q. "You don't know whether the sperm which you found was that of a Negro or a white man, do you?"

A. "There is no way of telling that, sir."

Mr. Johnson: "Thank you; that's all."

Among the series of questions I had submitted to Arthur Kinoy for possible exploration at the new trial were some relating to the proof of rape. Was the finding of sperm on the slide of the material taken from the alleged victim's body ever confirmed by an independent expert? (Other material on the slide could have been confused with sperm.) Was the ability of the physician who testified as to the finding of sperm ever substantiated in court? What was his previous experience in these matters? Was the slide available for evidence and review by an expert of defense counsel's choosing? Could the blood reported to be oozing from the alleged victim's womb have been merely the result of a normal menstrual flow? Lack of clear-cut answers to these few questions could raise serious doubts as to whether the act of rape had ever been committed.

Seal was imprisoned for about ten more years, while the legal battle was fought in his behalf. He is now free.

I didn't hear from Kinoy again until four years later, in August 1964. He called to find out if I would go to Mississippi to witness the autopsies of Goodman, Schwerner, and Chaney. "It may turn out to be a wild-goose chase," he said, "but you never know what will turn up. It's best to leave nothing to chance."

In the summer of 1964, hundreds of idealistic white students had joined with the rising new breed of militant but non-violent black youth in a unified effort to break open Mississippi's medieval, closed society. The campaign's main thrust was voter registration. The students were the shock troops, and in the rear—supplying legal, medical, moral, and financial needs—were lawyers, doctors, nurses, church groups, and other interested persons. Among these youthful missionaries, and working together as a unit, were Andrew Goodman, white, age twenty, Queens College student; Michael Schwerner, white, age twenty-four, Colgate graduate and social worker; and James Chaney, black, age twenty-one, a Catholic parochial-school dropout from Mississippi. While on one of their missions, they were reported missing, and the news flashed across the country. The nation waited and watched. If the pattern of the years held true, the civil-rights workers were most certainly dead. But only the killers and the ones to whom they boasted knew the facts. As the days went by, only their parents and close friends clung to any hope that they were still alive.

The blue Ford station wagon in which the three civil-rights workers had been traveling was found charred and burned along a road ten miles northeast of Philadelphia, Mississippi. This gruesome discovery intensified the search.

The FBI moved into action.

Mississippi Governor Paul Johnson said this could happen anywhere, and he was "satisfied" that everything possible was being done to locate the three civil-rights workers, now missing for a week.

On July 22, about three weeks later, Senator Eastland cynically suggested that the disappearance of these civil-rights workers in Mississippi might have been a hoax. He questioned charges that the three had been killed. In Philadelphia Deputy Sheriff Rainey refused to join in the search.

On August 3 (after the FBI produced a sworn statement by a paid informer that the bodies were buried there), a federal judge in Biloxi authorized the FBI to enter the Burrage farm, the site of a twenty-foot-high clay dam.

A bulldozer and FBI agents with shovels uncovered a "cruel tomb," eighteen feet beneath the surface of this clay dam. The remains of the three bodies were placed in plastic bags tagged X1, X2, and X3. Later, at the morgue of the University of Mississippi Medical School Hospital, in Jackson, the bodies were identified. The unofficial reports to the newspapers stated that Schwerner and Goodman had each been shot once in the chest and that Chaney had been shot several times.

Louis Lomax, black author and lecturer, was at the scene. He reported the words of one Negro Mississippian: "I am sorry that these fellows is dead. But five of us that we know about have been killed this year, and nobody raised hell about it. This time they killed two ofays. Now two white boys is dead and all the world come running to look and see. They never would have done this had just us been dead."

I was at our summer home on Martha's Vineyard when I got the second call. The phone rang about 1:30 A.M. I had just gone to sleep, after a restless hour in bed contemplating four days of utter failure to get my outboard motor running, and I walked half asleep down the dark hallway to the telephone, certain that it was a wrong number. The phone doesn't ring too often out there.

The operator said that Jackson, Mississippi, was calling.

The man on the wire was Dr. Charles Goodrich, a New York physician who was spending his vacation in Mississippi giving medical aid to the civil-rights workers as a volunteer for the Medical Committee for Human Rights.

"Dr. Spain, can you get down here right away?"

"To Mississippi?"

"Immediately. The autopsy for those three kids is scheduled for tomorrow, and the attorneys for Mrs. Chaney and Mickey Schwerner's family want an expert pathologist at the examination as an independent observer."

Goodrich said he had verbal permission for me to observe the autopsy. People in New York were working on a way to get me from the little island off the coast of Massachusetts to Mississippi by lunchtime. "You find a way to get me there, and I'll go," I said.

Then I went back to bed and waited.

At 3:00 A.M., the phone rang again. There is a small airport on Martha's Vineyard. I was to be there at 7:00 A.M. A special plane would take me to Kennedy International, where I could catch a 9:15 flight to Mississippi that would get me into Jackson fifteen minutes before the autopsy was scheduled to begin.

When I went back to sleep this time, I had forgotten about my outboard motor.

It was still dark when we got up and my wife drove me to the airstrip. But there was no small plane. Instead we got a phone call from the pilot. He couldn't get his motor started. I told him I knew just how he felt and put in a call to Jackson to tell Goodrich that things looked pretty hopeless. The only scheduled flight from the island into Kennedy was at ten, too late to make the morning plane to Mississippi, and the next flight for Jackson left at four in the afternoon from Newark Airport.

As I waited in the telephone booth for the operator to get through, my feelings were mixed. I was relieved at not having to interrupt my vacation, and I hadn't particularly looked forward to the reception an alien white man can get in Mississippi. But I was disappointed too, because I wouldn't have a chance now to do something that might help find the murderers of those kids. Goodrich, when he came on the phone, resolved my ambivalent feelings for me.

"Get down here anyway. Take the late plane. There's something funny going on about this business. I think we may be able to arrange for you to examine the bodies later. It may all be a wild-goose chase, but let's try."

I said good-by and then told my wife that I was going to Mississippi after all.

I had eight minutes to spare at Kennedy Airport before catching a helicopter to Newark, so I talked a barber into giving me perhaps what is the fastest haircut on the books. I saw myself in the barber-shop mirror and cried a little. My vacation wardrobe at Martha's Vineyard consisted of an eclectic assortment of well-broken-in loafing clothes, and I had dressed for my mission to Mississippi in battered suntans, a sport shirt, and a faded blue-denim sailing jacket. In a burst of insecurity, I had the bootblack shine my shoes. On the way out, I bought a white shirt and tie and put them on, which provided a dapper foil to my dirty tans and denim jacket. I could guess what proper Mississippians would think of the "medical examiner from the East."

The Newark plane left on time, and I had just unfastened my seatbelt when I heard a man across the aisle tell the stewardess to let him know if "you run across anybody named Spain." I answered up, and he introduced himself as Dr. Aaron Wells, the Chairman of the Medical Committee for Human Rights. He was traveling, by coincidence, on the same plane and had heard from Dr. Goodrich that I might be aboard. I moved across the aisle so we could chat, and we soon became good friends. Dr.

Wells, an assistant professor of medicine at Cornell, was one of the organizers of the medical committee, which was set up on an emergency basis when physical violence became standard operating procedure against civil-rights workers in Mississippi. The committee sent over one hundred doctors and nurses to work in the South that summer, and it is now a permanent volunteer organization. The committee, Wells said, was expanding its operations beyond medical care to a study of the effect of discrimination on the health of Southern Negroes, an investigation of cases where federal funds might be used in segregated medical facilities, and a survey of the public-health problems of Negroes—something largely neglected in the South.

The plane made a scheduled stop at Birmingham, and the stewardess soon came down the aisle and told us that one of the engines wouldn't turn over for the takeoff and there would be an indefinite delay. Dr. Wells and I went out for dinner.

The restaurant in the Birmingham airport is modern and attractive and I suggested we try it. Dr. Wells hesitated. "Do you think it's wise?" he said. "Do you think it will be OK?"

Dr. Wells is a Negro.

I found myself embarrassed at his embarrassment, and I said that airports were now legally desegregated, so I didn't think there'd be any trouble. Our uneasiness ebbed away after a couple of drinks and a good dinner. The waitress, who spoke in a syrupy southern drawl, was extremely gracious and attentive, and as we got back onto the plane I began to wonder if my preconceptions about the South might be a lot worse than the reality. It didn't take long in Jackson to find out that they weren't.

It was dark when we landed at the Jackson airport. I suggested that we take a cab to the hotel, but Dr. Wells said, very quietly, "No, I don't think we'd better." I looked at him and I saw in the pain and fear and dignity in his eyes what he meant without his saying anything further: After dark in Mississippi, it is poison for a Negro and a white person to be seen on the streets together. It is doubtful that there was a cab driver in the city who would have dared to pick us up. Dr. Wells called the medical committee headquarters, and a car was sent out for us.

We were driven to the Sun and Sands, a modern, glass-front hotel with a central patio and pool; it was desegregated and a frequent stopping place for representatives of civil-rights organizations.

I got my first hate stare in the lobby. The stare is an almost instinctive reaction of Mississippians who see a white man, especially a "foreign" white man, with a Negro. My felony was compounded because I asked for a room with one. Dr. Wells had planned to spend that night with a local Negro minister, but when we got into town after dark I suggested that he stay with me. When I told the girl behind the desk I wanted a room for two, her head snapped back as if I had jabbed the ball-point registration pen into her stomach.

"You two?" she asked. Her voice was a tempered mixture of incredulity and disgust.

I finished filling out the registration card. Her hand hit the page for the bellboy as if the metal bell were a slug she was trying to brush away.

The first thing Dr. Wells said after the bellboy left the room was, "What do you think is the best thing to do if somebody throws a bomb in the room?" He said it very seriously, and it took me a few seconds to realize that he wasn't kidding. "Do you think we should run, or try to throw the thing out before it goes off? I've been thinking about this for some time," he said. I said that I had no experience with anything like that, but that I imagined it would be best to run into the next room. As I answered him, I found myself wondering at the sound of my own words—wondering what kind of a never-never world we were in that we were seriously discussing bombs.

Dr. Goodrich called and asked us to come down to the room of John Pratt, an upstate New York attorney who was representing the Lawyers Constitutional Defense Committee in Jackson. Pratt was handling the arrangements for the autopsy. I wasn't prepared for the scene in Pratt's room.

When the door shut, I thought I was inside the headquarters of a battle battalion. Pratt's small room seemed filled with people—I counted at least ten—all moving and talking at the same frantic pace. One young man was in a serious phone conversation, another was pacing the floor, several others were studying documents that looked like legal briefs, and some others picked in lackluster fashion at food that had apparently just been brought in. Three men suddenly rushed out the front door, and it had barely closed when two other men and a girl came in. Pratt was in the middle of all this consternation, a tall, wiry man in his early thirties, talking, laughing occasionally, issuing instructions, and occasionally taking a bite out of a cold baked potato sitting in lonely splendor on a plate on top of the bureau.

The girl walked up to me. She was pretty, barely into her twenties, and looked as though she might have been out cheering the Beatles the night before. There was no smile on her face, and her voice was even and emotionless.

"Here is your orientation packet, Dr. Spain." She handed me a large manila envelope. It was given to all volunteers who came into Mississippi. I read the papers inside with a growing sense of uneasiness. An "orientation sheet" listed typical problems civil-rights volunteers encountered in Mississippi and suggestions to avoid them. One page was a memorandum of various psychological problems that some civil-rights workers faced—such as the need of some whites to mentally "become a Negro" before they could adjust to working there, or the tensions and misunderstandings that at times developed between white men and Negro women, and vice versa, who worked together.

There was also a list entitled "Security Regulations." I was to always let committee people know where I was going, was not to be out on the streets alone at night, and should report my whereabouts to headquarters every three hours when I was away from the hotel.

The girl gave me a list of phone numbers to call if I was arrested ("You might be arrested at any time that you're on the streets"), and asked me for a friend they could call if I had to make bail.

Then, for the first time, I felt the full shock of the monstrous implications of what was happening in Mississippi. Up until this time, I was thinking of the trip, though made under extraordinary circumstances, as just another assignment. Suddenly I had an entirely different perspective. It was hard to rationalize the possibility that I could be arrested, that I might be in physical danger—just because I was in Mississippi. It was like being in the middle of a war game—only, the other side was shooting real bullets.

Pratt briefed me on the situation. He had been trying frantically to get permission for me to examine the bodies but had met one legal roadblock after another. The official post-mortem examination had been made that afternoon, but the authorities decided not to allow any independent observers as witnesses. Pratt's staff spent the day gathering all the affidavits and notarized documents that the authorities required for permission to examine the bodies—but each time they filled one request, another took its place.

Pratt was forced to take a heart-burdening step. He asked Mrs. Chaney, the mother of one of the slain boys, for permission to have her son's body examined by me as soon as the body was released to her by the authorities. She agreed without any hesitation. The Neshoba County district attorney then promised Pratt that when all papers were in order he would sanction the release of the body to Mrs. Chaney and we could get on with our grim task.

Finally, at 1:00 A.M., the last of the legal papers was stacked neatly on Pratt's desk. All that was left to do was call the district attorney and have him authorize the director of the University of Mississippi Hospital, where the autopsy had been performed, to release the body of James Chaney to Mrs. Chaney and to us for examination. The district attorney, Raiford Jones, had given Pratt his home telephone number. Pratt put in a call to the DA. When he put down the receiver a few minutes later, his thin face was hot with frustration.

"The operator says the DA's phone is out of order and will be out of order for twenty-four hours."

Pratt asked the police in Philadelphia, where Jones lives, to go out to his house and deliver the message. He made the request halfheartedly. The police didn't call back.

Before I went to bed, I read carefully the accounts in the late newspapers of the post-mortem examination that had been made on the boys that afternoon. The examination was conducted, the story said, by a private pathologist ostensibly appointed by the coroner, the University of Mississippi Pathology Department, and the FBI. The report said that the bodies were badly decomposed, that all three boys had been shot, Schwerner and Goodman once and Chaney three times, and that there was no other evidence of mutilation or bodily injury. It also said that Chaney's wrist had been fractured by a bullet.

This report was quickly dispatched by the wire services. The impression given nationally was that a meticulous examination had been made of the deceased under the supervision of university pathologists and the FBI. But the report just didn't make good medical sense to me. The statements that the bodies were badly decomposed and that there was no evidence of mutilation or other injury were contradictory: if the bodies were badly decomposed, it would be extremely unlikely that an official determination could be made as to the extent of bodily injuries. The maddening technicalities that kept me from examining the bodies left me angry. I began, in a solemn mood, to look forward to my sad task the next day.

Dr. Wells and I went down to the hotel dining room for breakfast the next morning. The hostess sat us at a table directly in front of the door, and after some discussion she reluctantly moved us farther inside the dining room. That, I guess, was a mistake. The table next to us sagged under a giant, weighing somewhere between 300 and 350 pounds, with a bright-red sunburnt neck the breadth of a miniature saddle. He was hunched over the table, which was heaped with a fantastic assortment of food, which I believe represented every entree on the breakfast menu: stacked pancakes, ham, several fried eggs, sausages, hominy grits, hashed brown potatoes—and a medium-sized breakfast steak.

Both his hands were moving at the same time toward his mouth in a remarkable exhibition of physical co-ordination. Between shovels, he happened to glance over at our table. He was thunderstruck. His hands hung, motionless, in mid-air. He stopped chewing. He stared at us in complete disbelief. He seemed unable to comprehend that a white man and a Negro were actually sitting together at a table across from him. He jerked his thick neck down toward the plate and tried to go back to his food, but he couldn't stop staring at us. He would concentrate on eating, and almost immediately his head would snap back in our direction. This went on for at least ten minutes, with his head snapping up and down as if he were watching an indoor tennis match. His hate stares were directed at me— his eyes were signposts saying HATE—I was a white man betraying his race because I was having breakfast with a black man. The "redneck" (this is, curiously, a slang term in the South for White Citizens Council types; in this case, it was also a physical description) finally gave up the uneven match with his attention and pushed back his chair like the Queen Mary leaving berth. He sidled out of the dining room.

I realize this man sounds like a caricature. But he was real. This is one of the incredible things about Mississippi: caricature is real.

Dr. Wells left for the medical committee headquarters, and I walked out into the center patio and found John Pratt sitting in a deck chair beside the pool.

"Sit down," he said. "There's nothing to do now but wait."

The funeral director hired by Mrs. Chaney was on his way to Philadelphia, Pratt said, with all the papers necessary to effect the release of young Chaney's body. After presenting the papers to the Philadelphia authorities, he would drive back to Jackson, stop at the hotel for us, and then proceed to the University of Mississippi Medical Center, where I could examine Chaney. The round trip would take about five hours, so we had nothing to do but wait until he showed up.

In the meantime, two COFO (Council of Federated Organizations, a broad front of civil-rights groups) workers had taken up positions at the morgue entrance to make sure the bodies would not be removed without our knowledge.

In retrospect, it seems amazing how you can proceed with the ordinary pleasures of life in the midst of such a situation, but that is what we did. We went swimming, sunned ourselves at poolside, and chatted. The conversation was almost light-hearted—a reaction, I think, against contemplating the grim job before us.

I told Pratt that I had brought a book with me: *Mississippi: The Closed Society*. Pratt frowned. "If you plan to read that in the open, out here at the pool, I suggest you take off the dust jacket. These people around here are pretty touchy—they don't like outsiders reading about them." I must admit that I felt rather silly, removing the jacket of my book. But I did it. I had decided to take the advice of Mississippi veterans on the best way to survive in that strange country.

I became aware that there were no Negroes in the pool. I asked Pratt what would happen if a Negro guest of this desegregated hotel went swimming.

"Oh, it's been tried," Pratt said. "But something always happens—like the hotel management suddenly announcing that the filter system is 'not functioning properly' and it is necessary to clear the pool for an indefinite period of time. The word gets around quick enough to the Negroes, and as far as I know, no Negro has ever succeeded in swimming one lap in that pool."

"How did Mrs. Chaney take it—when you talked to her about examining her son's body?"

I asked a question that had been in my mind since I had heard about the bereaved mother's brave decision consenting to a second autopsy on her son.

"She was beautiful," Pratt said. "When I asked her, she said, very quietly, 'I want everyone to know everything possible about what has happened.' Then she added: 'I know he could die only once, but if they did these awful things to him, this ought to be no secret. It is even more important now that the guilty ones be brought to trial and justice and be punished. God must forgive them; it is very difficult for me to do so.' "

The pressure on Mrs. Chaney to refuse permission was tremendous: Philadelphia—white Philadelphia, that is—was against it. Without her, we would never see the body; the authorities in Philadelphia seemed decidedly unfavorable to a second medical examination. "Philadelphia is like an armed camp," Pratt said. "When I went there to see the district attorney, he had to arrange for me to arrive in the city incognito. Unemployed white men—they're called "deputy sheriffs" in Philadelphia—strut around the center of town all day, displaying their gun holsters, on the watch for any "intruders." The atmosphere is murderous. Mrs. Chaney's a widow with young children. It took a lot of guts for her to sign those papers. Retaliation is easy in Philadelphia." And so it was. Three weeks later, Mrs. Chaney's home was bombed and shot into.

Pratt was paged on the hotel public-address system. When he went inside to answer the phone, I browsed through a file of reports from field teams of the Medical Committee for Human Rights. I had the stomach to read only two of them.

The first report described extended treatment given a young Negro civil-rights worker for fifteen or twenty burns scattered all over his body. He had been stopped by the police in a small Mississippi town for questioning, and while they questioned him they jabbed lighted cigarettes into his flesh. The burns weren't treated, and were ulcerous and infected when the medical volunteers found him.

Another Mississippi town, a medical report said, had activated a local statute requiring any "stranger" entering the town to register at police headquarters—as if he were entering a foreign country. The youth in the report had registered, but a policeman had insisted that the boy come to the station to "check" his compliance with the statute. The boy's name was found on the books. The officer then told him to "run along," and in the same breath swung his billy club into the boy's groin with such force that the youth passed out. Surgery was later necessary to evacuate a blood clot (larger than an orange) created by the blow.

I was too depressed to read further. I have no reason to doubt the authenticity of these reports. After conversations with physicians who have been in Mississippi, I believe that incidents of this nature—with varying degrees of brutality—went on regularly and relentlessly every day of the week. They were too frequent to be considered "newsworthy."

In the rarefied atmosphere of Mississippi, the grotesque becomes matter of fact, and the simplest idea can meet the strangest and most insurmountable obstacles. One pitifully sad case in point: Mickey Schwerner's parents and James Chaney's mother decided that they would like both their sons buried together in the Chaney family plot in Mississippi. This just couldn't be done. The Negro funeral director for Mrs. Chaney did not dare to pick up the white boy's body at the University Hospital. If he did, he feared some technical reason would be found for revoking his license. And the bereaved Schwerners were unable to find a white undertaker in Mississippi who would transport the body of their son to a Negro cemetery. They were forced to abandon the idea.

Pratt came in and said that our wait was over. The undertaker had arrived with the necessary papers. Dr. Wells, Dr. Goodrich, Mr. Pratt, and I drove together to the morgue. As we passed through the quiet and clean streets of Jackson, I was hit by the horrible realization that this pleasant town—the opposite of the stereotype of the "typical" southern town, with nary a Faulknerian degenerate ghosting the streets—was actually a façade. The scary thing was that Jackson looked so pleasant and sleepy—and if this rotten core of hate could be underneath, it could be anywhere.

Our official reception at the morgue was cool, but courteous. The University of Mississippi Medical Center is a large and striking building in downtown Jackson, built, incidentally, with federal funds. We met the director of the hospital and several members of the pathology department in the well-lit basement hallway that leads to the autopsy room. We exchanged professional courtesies, and one of the doctors pointed toward the double stainless-steel doors ahead of us. "It's inside," he said.

Only two of the bodies were still there. Goodman's corpse had been sent out the night before, and he was buried before there was a chance for a second autopsy. The Mississippi authorities refused to allow Schwerner's parents to give telephone permission for me to examine the body—so it was young Chaney who lay on the gurney wheeled to the center of the room.

One of the university pathologists stepped forward silently and helped me slide Chaney's corpse from the gurney to the stainless-steel examining table in the middle of the room. He stepped backward and lined up with his two comrades on one side of the table, facing me. I stood alone on the opposite side. The only sound in the room was the rough noise of the zipper on the protective plastic bag as I pulled it away from Chaney's body.

I was immediately struck by how slight and frail this young man was—a thin boy with tender skin. I looked at his wrist, the one that was reported broken in the official examination, and I couldn't find the bullet hole that the newspapers had mentioned. The wrist was certainly broken. Bones were smashed, so badly that his wrist must have literally flapped. But there was no indication of any bullet hole. I looked up at the three doctors opposite me. Their faces were stone. I motioned to the wrist. I asked where the bullet hole was. One of the stone figures facing me offered a mumbled explanation, something about how Chaney's hand had been across his chest when the first examination was made and the examiner must have mistaken the bullet holes in his chest for one in the hand. I looked at him in amazement, but our eyes never met. During the remainder of the examination, not another word was spoken.

Then I noticed Chaney's jaw. It was broken: the lower jaw was completely shattered, split vertically, from some tremendous force. I moved the shattered pieces of his jaw in vertical directions for the three doctors to see. They remained silent. I couldn't catch their eyes.

I carefully examined the body and found that the bones in the right shoulder were crushed—again, from some strong and direct blow. His internal organs had been removed in the first autopsy, so it was impossible to ascertain if Chaney had suffered internal injuries also.

But one thing was certain: this frail boy had been beaten in an unhuman fashion. The blows that had so terribly shattered his bones—I surmised he must have been beaten with chains, or a pipe—were in themselves sufficient to cause death. It was again impossible to say if he had died before he was shot: the bullets had been removed in the first autopsy, and the bullet tracks had been carefully excised so I could not trace the paths of the bullets.

I examined the skull, and it was crushed too. The fracture was circular and depressed, from another direct blow. I could scarcely believe the destruction to these frail young bones. In my thirty years as a pathologist and medical examiner, I have never seen bones so severely shattered, except in tremendously high-speed accidents or airplane crashes. It was obvious to any first-year medical student that this boy had been beaten to a pulp. I found myself so emotionally charged that it was difficult for me to retain my professional composure. I felt every fiber in my own body shaking, as I imagined the scene at the time this youngster received a beating so vicious as to shatter his bones in this incredible manner.

I wanted to scream at these impassive observers silently standing across the table. But I knew my rage would not penetrate their curtain of silence. I took off the green surgical smock they had given me, thanked them for their co-operation, and left the room as quickly as I could. I returned to the hotel, dictated a report of my gruesome findings, and left immediately for the airport.

I felt an obsessive urge to get out of Mississippi the fastest way possible. The first plane out went the wrong way to New York—to New Orleans—but I felt indescribable relief when I boarded it and flew—I guess you could say I fled—from Jackson.

Back home, the news of my findings, reported widely in the press, had preceded my return. I had been in Mississippi for only twenty-four hours, never in danger, doing a small job for which I had been previously trained. Yet, upon my return, some of the "movement" people regarded me as some sort of minor hero or celebrity. Unfortunately all movements seem to need a steady diet of "more or less" heroes; most, as I, are unauthentic; and sooner or later they all are devoured. I have found very few long-distance runners, perhaps because it is too lonely, or else because they become victims of their own television image.

Maxwell Geismar, the literary historian and biographer, suggested I write a brief account of my twenty-four-hour experience. It was published in *Ramparts*. I was deluged with requests to speak on behalf of the co-ordinating council of the civil-rights organizations at various church groups, temples, and many civil-rights meetings. There was a flurry of television and radio interviews, an appearance on the David Susskind show, and even one nightclub appearance moderated by Betty Furness.

My world had changed. Civil-rights pathology had sadly come of age.

Months later, there was still no official report or word from Mississippi. The blackout was total. Finally, on July 5, 1965, the silence was unofficially broken. I received a letter from Professor Louis Lasagna, of Johns Hopkins University. It contained a copy of a letter sent to him by one of Mississippi's leading pathologists. He was exercized by an article Dr. Lasagna had written, entitled "Physicians and the Macrocosm," which appeared in the April 1965 issue of the *Yale Journal of Biology and Medicine*. This pathologist was offended by a statement in Lasagna's article making "unflattering comparisons" between Mississippi physicians and the Nazis.

Since Dr. Lasagna had made reference to the article I'd written for *Ramparts,* much of the pathologist's ire was directed at me. He claimed that I had no right to form any conclusions, since I hadn't seen the official autopsy report and had not autopsied the bodies but only made a "casual five minute external examination" of one body. He indicated that the fractures I believed had occurred because of a beating might have occurred *after* death—that the bulldozers that uncovered the graves might have either run over or dropped the bodies. He closed by saying that he had "little confidence" in my ability to remember things accurately, since I had remembered the tiles in the autopsy room to be green, and there are, according to him, no green tiles there. I suppose it is my own fault for trying to play interior decorator; nevertheless, I would have thought it obvious that a professional can have total recall in his field without being especially observant in other, non-related fields.

I prepared a detailed rebuttal for Dr. Lasagna of these and the other points the Mississippi pathologist made in his letter. For example, despite the allegation that I didn't really examine the bodies, I examined two of the three. I performed a complete autopsy on Mr. Schwerner in Brooklyn at the I. J. Morris Funeral Home on August 10, 1964, with four witnesses in attendance. I examined what was left of Mr. Chaney in Jackson, Mississippi—and there wasn't much left except the skeleton and the skin. The internal organs had been removed and thrown away. I was afraid to make an incision in the body; my northerner's paranoia told me that if I did, I would be charged with performance of an autopsy in a state where I was not licensed to practice medicine. I did what I could within the limits of the body as it was.

I did not base my conclusions on the official autopsy report, because there *was* none. The only report issued by official sources was the Neshoba County coroner's report, after a delay of a number of months (it usually is just a matter of days), and all it said was that cause of death could not be determined. To this day, nine years after the autopsies, an official autopsy report has not been made public.

As for the fascinating suggestion that the fractures I noticed might have been made by a bulldozer: To the best of my knowledge, the fractures were only present in the body of the black youth. How a bulldozer managed to mangle him without damaging the two white bodies is beyond me; I am more persuaded that the black body was beaten, and the whites not, for the same reason that the black body had three bullet wounds and the whites only one apiece. Overkill, I think it's called. I cannot conceive of any bulldozer or any fall that could account for the fractures I saw. I challenged this pathologist, in my rebuttal, to set up a satisfactory, concrete set of circumstances, even a theoretical model, of how the injuries could have happened as he suggested. I have received no answer from him.

A discrepancy in the pathologist's letter caught my attention. He claimed that four pathologists performed the "autopsies" on the three bodies. In actual fact, I found, upon examining Mr. Schwerner's body, that no complete autopsy had actually been performed. The only thing that had been done was a chest incision to remove the bullet from the body, but there had not been a full autopsy as reasonable men understand the term. I didn't see Andrew Goodman's body, but there had not been detailed autopsies on all three. I also don't believe there were four men constantly present at the Chaney autopsy, and I base my belief on the words of the three members of the University of Mississippi Pathology Department, whom I assume were three of the alleged "four." When I arrived at the university morgue, I asked these men who had performed the autopsy on Chaney. They informed me that Dr. Featherstone, a local pathologist, had performed the autopsy on behalf of the coroner. "We really didn't see the entire autopsy," one of them told me, "because we were in and out of the room."

My correspondent also denigrated the validity of my findings because I had published in a lay magazine instead of a scientific journal. This is what I wrote in reply:

"I have tried to be objective, but in reality this is not entirely an objective answer. Whatever the value of objectivity—and we can certainly enumerate these values with appreciation—it is not a condition which should be raised to a way of life. Life is for living—it is not for looking at or being disposed to. Science is made for man—not man for Science. It is for this latter reason that the distinction that was made between lay magazines and scientific journals has no validity in this situation. This is not merely a technological question. It is a deeply human one."

I am aware that my response, composed in the heat of anger, contained elements of a stultifying moral self-righteousness. With a detachment cooled by the passage of time, I understand that in like circumstances I, too, fearful of my surroundings and for my future, might react similarly. No doubt these men of whom I have spoken are ordinarily sensitive, good, and innately ethical. That is, of course, all the more distressing—that decent citizens can accept not only prejudice but murder itself in the defense of prejudice.

One gets to the kind of slanted views I have described through small steps. It can begin with the small and seemingly insignificant act of substituting the lower case "n" for the capital "N" in "Negro" wherever it appears in scientific papers. The next step is taken when scientists in a recognized medical publication claim that there is a higher death rate for blacks receiving anesthetics because of their "inferior central nervous system." In actuality, there is well-established scientific evidence that 1) the heavier pigmentation of blacks masks the early development of cyanosis—lips turning blue—which would warn an anesthesiologist that there is trouble; and 2) doctors often fail to uncover a sickle-cell trait, a disease found almost only in Negroes which tends to block oxygen supply to the blood. The corrosive effects of racism can, in this fashion, distort professional integrity and reason.

Ever since the murders, it had been common knowledge in and around Philadelphia who had committed the crimes. The men couldn't be tried for murder, since the coroner never officially determined the cause of death. They were finally brought to trial under a federal law for violating the civil rights of their three victims, and received short jail sentences on their conviction.

Some good resulted from this tragedy. I do not think that such a crime will ever again go unscrutinized, undisclosed, and unresolved.

3. MURDER AND JUSTICE CHICAGO STYLE—THE CASE OF FRED HAMPTON

The beast must die, also the man.

Ecclesiasticus

The colorless prose of legal documents makes even the most controversial case sound dull. When Fred Hampton, deputy chairman of the Black Panther Party, was shot and killed in Chicago, this is what the federal grand jury had to say about it:

"At 4:45 A.M., December 4, 1969, fourteen Chicago Police officers assigned to the Cook County States Attorney's Office executed a search warrant for illegal weapons at 2337 West Monroe Street in a flat rented by members of the Black Panther Party. Nine people were in the apartment. Two were killed in the gunfire which broke out: Fred Hampton, the militant and controversial chairman of the Black Panther Party of Illinois, and Mark Clark, a Panther official from Peoria. Four occupants were wounded, but survived. Two police officers sustained minor injuries."

Some additional facts not mentioned by the grand jury report add flesh to these bare bones: The squad of fourteen policemen

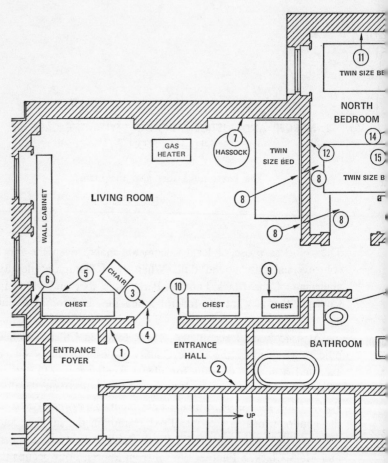

The police version: In the shoot-out, Hampton was hit by bullets coming through the wall and was found dead on his stomach. The numbers show bullet holes.

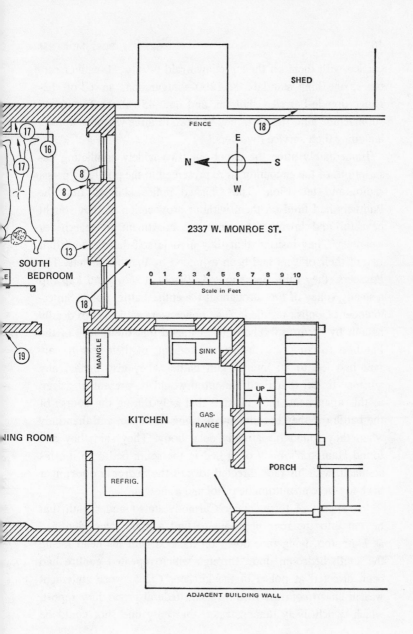

SHED

FENCE

⑱

E
N ◄ ⊕ S
W

2337 W. MONROE ST.

0 1 2 3 4 5 6 7 8 9 10
Scale in Feet

⑰
⑯
⑰
⑧
⑧
⑬
SOUTH
BEDROOM
⑱
⑲

MANGLE
SINK

UP

KITCHEN
GAS-
RANGE

DINING ROOM

REFRIG.

PORCH

ADJACENT BUILDING WALL

carried with them on their predawn raid twenty .30-caliber car-
bines, one high standard K 1200 shotgun, one sawed-off 12-
gauge double-barreled shotgun, and one .45-caliber Thompson
submachine gun. In short, they had two to three weapons apiece,
including their service revolvers.

Immediately after the shoot-out, two widely conflicting descriptions of the encounter were presented to the public by press,
radio, and television. The Chicago police claimed that the
Panthers had fired on them without provocation as they sought
peaceful and lawful entry into the apartment to search for
weapons. They insisted that they fired in self-defense and that
two of their officers had been wounded by Panther bullets. The
Panthers, they said, had shouted, "Shoot it out," and kept up
a steady volley of fire throughout the entire battle. Police Super-
intendent Conlisk testified, "The police were subjected to deadly
assault by firearms." The police claimed that the failure of the
Panthers to comply with the requirements of their search warrant had led to an intense gun battle. They also denied any
advance tip-off that Fred Hampton would be present or asleep
in this apartment; they insisted that only during the course of
the battle did they become aware of his presence, and then only
when they found his already dead body. They said they had
found Hampton's body on a bed in the south bedroom, on his
stomach, with his face directed toward the bedroom door; near
his body were an automatic pistol and a shotgun.

In support of this, Officer Carmody stated under oath that
he ran into the rear bedroom to find a man, later identified
as Hampton, lying face down on the bed with his head facing
the south bedroom door, through which repeated gunfire had
been directed at police in the kitchen. (This sworn statement
was in sharp contrast to the official federal grand jury report,
which conclusively demonstrated that only one shot could be

proved to have come from a Panther gun—and this shot had not originated from the south bedroom.)

Spokesmen for the Black Panthers flatly denied this story; they charged that the police version was a complete fabrication, and counterclaimed that Hampton and Clark were victims of a Chicago-style political assassination. They claimed that, following the struggle, there was tangible physical evidence in the apartment that unequivocally showed that the police, without any warning to the occupants, had fired first and had continued to shoot despite the lack of any overt resistance. They also disputed the police description of the positioning of Fred Hampton's body: They charged that Hampton had been deliberately killed in his sleep while lying on his back. Although they agreed that his head had been at the end of the bed toward the door, they claimed that his face had been directed toward the other end of the bed, away from the bedroom door. He had been lying in a defenseless position, they said, and had not engaged in any shoot-out, as the police had implied. Hampton's wife said she'd been sleeping in bed with him when the shooting started; she had run out of the room, but he hadn't moved.

Later that day, on December 4, 1969, the body of Fred Hampton was autopsied by a pathologist of the Cook County coroner's office at the Institute of Forensic Medicine. The Chicago coroner's autopsy concluded that Fred Hampton had been shot four times and seemed to back up the police report that Hampton had been on his stomach. According to the autopsy report, one bullet had proceeded at an angle from left to right, entering the head in front of the left ear and exiting from the right forehead. A second bullet had entered the right side of the neck, two inches below the bottom of the right earlobe, proceeding also at an angle from right to left and exiting from the left side of the throat. A left-shoulder bullet-wound track led to a .30-caliber carbine bullet that was found embedded in the left front chest muscles. A fourth bullet was said to have grazed the skin of the right forearm. It was deduced from these findings that the bullets striking Hampton had come from several directions, as described by the police at the time of the raid. Surprisingly, the coroner's pathologist took no pictures of the bullet wounds. Only identification photographs were available, and these were useless for a study of the wounds.

The failure to document the wounds with close-up photographs in a case of such national prominence mystified me. In all modern medical examiners' offices and even, with rare exception, in most old-fashioned coroners' departments, photography is an essential and routine procedure in all homicides. Where the pathologist does not have the facilities for photography, the local law-enforcement agencies invariably provide police photographers, who carefully record all of the wounds. When I was retained by the father of Raymond Lavon Moore in the Tomb's suicide case, I performed a reautopsy in a small funeral parlor in an upstate New York town. We hired a local police photographer to record all of my findings in detail. Experience has shown that it is frequently possible, even with the most competent observers and with the most honest of intentions, to produce slight errors in drawn sketches and written descriptions of the measurements, location, and direction of bullet wounds in the body. These seemingly insignificant deviations sometimes can be crucial and produce important distortions in the true trajectory and direction of the bullets, leading to erroneous conclusions concerning the positions of the victim and the assailant. These errors may profoundly alter a proper interpretation of the findings and result in an injustice.

The most notorious recent example originated from such a distortion: the controversy over the origin and direction of the shots in the assassination of President Kennedy. This led to many books, articles, and debates, with all sorts of theories as to what had actually happened. Most, if not all, of the confusion and controversy could have been avoided if the Warren Commission's staff personnel had had access to the pictures and X rays taken at the autopsy. These clearly demonstrated that the initial bullet passed through John Kennedy's body at a distinctly downward angle, more than was shown on the schematic drawings released by the Warren Commission. The true angle of the path of the bullet virtually eliminated the possibility of this shot having been fired by someone hiding in the grassy knoll facing the President's car. It was this possibility that gave rise to the conspiracy theory (as opposed to the view that Oswald was the lone assassin).

The availability of clear pictorial documentation in courtroom testimony before a jury virtually eliminates any doubts about the accuracy of the observations or the integrity of the expert witness who is presenting this evidence. In the Hampton case, if such pictures were in reality not taken at the time of the initial autopsy, as was claimed under oath, it certainly has to be categorized as an act of incomprehensible carelessness or one of utter incompetence. If proper photographs had been available, the two later autopsies would have not been required and justice would have been served much sooner. Fortunately, despite this oversight it was eventually possible to rectify this glaring procedural omission.

On the day Hampton's body was first autopsied, and I would assume shortly thereafter, I received a phone call from Chicago. The voice appeared to be that of a teen-age girl. She introduced herself by giving her name and said she was a member of the Black Panther Party in Chicago. She asked if I would be willing and able to come to Chicago on behalf of her organization and reautopsy the body of their slain leader, Fred Hampton. These requests no longer surprised me. Ever since my visit to Mississippi in the summer of 1964, such inquiries have become, if not routine, at least almost commonplace events. And usually the caller has had little or no knowledge of the necessary legal preparation required to implement such a request. This was also the case even when the inquiries came from civil-rights lawyers. Surprisingly, and almost without exception, these attorneys were ignorant of the requirements that had to be fulfilled before a reautopsy could be performed. Of course, I did not expect this young girl to be aware of the procedure. I advised her to ask her legal counsel to contact me. That evening, Francis Andrew, one of the Panther lawyers, called to discuss the arrangements for a second post-mortem examination. He was now acting on behalf of Mrs. Hampton, Fred's mother. I suggested it might be more prudent to secure a Chicago-based pathologist and avoid the almost inevitable charges that a biased outsider (like me) was being brought into the case who could not possibly render an objective report. I had become sensitized to this problem several years before, in the Mississippi autopsy. The governor of that state had issued a statement to the press that in effect called me some sort of carpetbagger who had been brought into the great and sovereign state of Mississippi only to stir up trouble. After I assured Andrew that I would remain available in the event he failed to obtain a competent Chicago-based pathologist, he readily agreed to this proposal. I was not needed at this time, since Andrew was able to retain Dr. Victor Levine, former chief pathologist of the Chicago coroner's office. The choice of Dr. Levine was ideal, because he was locally based and had been a respected official. He was also in no way identified politically with the left or with the Black Panthers and could not be charged with having any prejudices in this situation.

That night, shortly after midnight, I was at a friend's home when another call came from Chicago, one that I almost subconsciously and humorously had been expecting and had become accustomed to. It was from the nationally known civil-rights

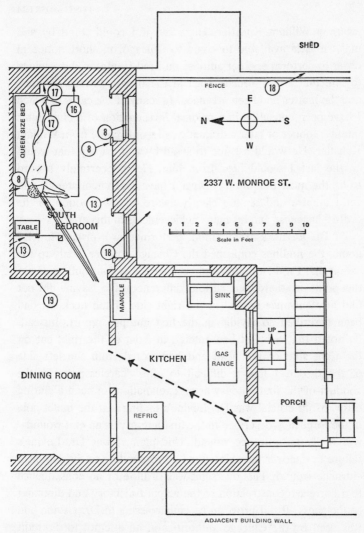

Position proved by the final autopsy: Hampton was lying on his side and was hit by four shots fired from the door. The Panthers claim some of the police entered through the kitchen.

attorney William Kunstler. He asked if I could stand by and
make myself available to come to Chicago on short notice in
order to perform another autopsy on Fred Hampton. I explained
to him that I had already been in touch with Francis Andrew
and the matter had been arranged. In many of the cases in which
I have been consulted in a medical investigation of a civil-rights
fatality, sooner or later a dramatic call would come from William
Kunstler. He would ask me to stand by and usually that would
be the last I would hear from him. He has certainly proved
to be the most ubiquitous lawyer I have ever encountered, and
yet I admire and remain clearly aware of his devotion to the
civil-rights cause and his many achievements in this area.

At Dr. Levine's examination, performed in a private funeral
home, the findings confirmed the Chicago coroner's only to the
extent that Fred Hampton had been struck by four bullets. From
this point on, there were serious differences. Dr. Levine did not
find any entrance wound in the right side of the neck, as had
been described so vividly in the first autopsy report. Instead,
he noted that a bullet had entered in front of the right ear on
the right side of the head and had exited from the left side
of the throat. I find it difficult to offer "carelessness" in the
conduct of the first autopsy as an explanation for such a glaring
error. More crucial was Dr. Levine's finding that the bullet hole
in the forehead—described in the first autopsy as an exit wound—
was really an entrance wound. Unexplained was Dr. Levine's
failure to uncover the exit wound corresponding to the forehead
entrance wound. This oversight was of little or no consequence
to a correct reconstruction of the actual trajectory and direction
of the shots. It did prove to be embarrassing to Dr. Levine and
was used by the Chicago authorities in an attempt to discredit
him. According to Dr. Levine, all the bullets seemed to have
entered or hit Hampton's body at about the same angle; they
had come from the right and proceeded in a slightly downward

direction, from right to left. Since, if he had been on his stomach, as the police claimed, the wall would have been on his right and the door on his left, these conclusions supported the Black Panthers' account of the position of Fred Hampton's body: lying on his back with the door at his right. At this second autopsy, all of the wounds were photographed in great detail. Enlarged reproductions and originals in 35mm. color photos were made available to me and are still in my possession.

The conflicting autopsy reports became one of the key public controversies surrounding the case.

Unfortunately, one element in the Levine reautopsy—a blood analysis—introduced a needless controversy into the case. The finding of a high level of seconal (a sleep-inducing drug), which was not found in the blood from the first autopsy, and disputed in another chemical examination at the FBI laboratories in Washington, served to confuse the issue and caused the Panthers to claim that Fred Hampton had been deliberately drugged by an inside agent of the police in order to render him defenseless during the planned attack.

Months afterward, in a conference with a commission of inquiry, I spent considerable time discussing the seconal question. Once raised, it had become a difficult matter to convince them that the finding was a spurious one, even though I had conducted my own analysis on the tissue obtained at the third autopsy and found it to be free of seconal. (I suspected that the lab technicians had simply misread their charts.) Hampton's defenders had become attracted to the theory that he had been drugged by an infiltrator from the police. The matter, from their point of view, was never completely put to rest.

The conflicting findings in the two autopsies aroused suspicions, naturally enough, especially in the black community. Black anger was intensified by photographs appearing in the Chicago *Tribune* that had been supplied by State's Attorney Edward V. Hanrahan. These pictures purported to show a hole in the living-room door of the raided apartment, allegedly from a bullet fired by the Panthers. A second picture was said to depict the inside of the bathroom door, showing many marks from shotgun pellets, also supposed to have been fired by the Panthers. Both these claims later proved to be false. The so-called shotgun-pellet holes were actually nailheads in the wood, and the Chicago *Sun-Times,* in an exposé, proved that the so-called closed living-room door was actually a door to the north bedroom and that the hole had resulted from a bullet fired by the police through the living-room wall.

These unsupported, erroneous, and perhaps fraudulent presentations prompted five separate citizens' groups to enter the controversy and pledge to investigate the situation: the Commission of Inquiry, headed by former Supreme Court Justice Arthur Goldberg and former Attorney General Ramsay Clark, consisting of twenty-six private citizens well known in the fields of civil rights, law, politics, and business; a delegation of black congressmen; the Chicago Afro-American Patrolmen's Association; the Black Strategy Center; and a people's inquest sponsored by the Black Panther Party.

Two Panthers had been killed and four had been wounded. None of the police had been injured by bullets or physical assault despite an earlier false claim to the contrary. In a meticulous search of the premises after the shoot-out, the FBI, Chicago police laboratory technicians, and trained crime investigators retained by the Black Panthers collectively examined and analyzed 188 spent bullets, shell casings, and shot shell components collected at the scene, and conclusively proved that the police had fired approximately one hundred shots and that only one shot could be positively identified as having been fired from a Black Panther weapon. Furthermore, this single shot, because of its point of origin, course, and point of impactation, was a highly questionable candidate for the opening shot of the foray. No wonder there was disbelief and dismay when on January 30, 1970, the Cook County grand jury not only absolved the police of any wrongdoing, but also handed down an indictment against the seven surviving occupants of the apartment charging them with attempt to commit murder and armed violence.

To abate the public outcry at these outrageous acts, the federal Department of Justice launched its own grand-jury inquiry. It soon became clear that any just determination required resolution of the conflicting findings of the two autopsies. The Justice Department, therefore, obtained a court order to exhume Hampton's body, buried in his birthplace, Shreveport, Louisiana.

Again I was called by Francis Andrew, and now I was retained to represent Mrs. Hampton as an observer at the third autopsy of her son. This required that I go to Shreveport.

Andrew and Mrs. Hampton, Fred's mother, had preceded me; they were staying at the home of Fred Hampton's aunt. Within a half hour of my arrival at the airport, they picked me up. Once in the car, I was introduced to Mrs. Hampton and her sister.

Mrs. Hampton impressed me by her calm but purposeful and determined approach to the entire affair. She told me that she had never believed in violence, but that she nevertheless understood what her son had been trying to do, and respected his single-minded devotion to the struggle "for the liberation of our people." She also expressed deep concern for Fred's child (recently born after Fred's death) and for her new grandson's mother.

At all times with the black mothers—Mrs. Chaney, Mrs. Hampton, and other parents of civil-rights victims—I always had a vague sense of not being trusted. If they on their part actually did not, it was never revealed by the slightest word or gesture.

I never mentioned this to anyone and tried to go about the business at hand in as compassionate and respectful a manner as the circumstances permitted.

The aunt's home was located in an all-black community of modest and well-cared-for homes. After serving us coffee and cake, Mrs. Hampton and her sister excused themselves and went shopping, but before leaving the house they warned it would be unwise for us to wander out in this neighborhood. After all, we could not walk around with signs on our backs proclaiming ourselves "good whities."

Francis Andrew and I reviewed documents and photographs of the previous autopsies, and the essential evidence relating to the circumstances surrounding the death, in order to be better prepared for the upcoming autopsy. Based on the available facts, we tried to construct the most plausible hypothesis of how Fred Hampton had been killed. At 3:30 P.M. we were driven to the local veterans hospital, where the examination was scheduled to take place.

At the hospital, Jerris Leonard, assistant attorney general, chief of the civil-rights section of the U. S. Justice Department, had arranged a briefing session to outline the ground rules for all the participants. Present were four representatives for the Illinois state's attorney's office (two assistant state's attorneys, Dr. Kearns of the Cook County coroner's office, and Dr. Mavrelis, a pathologist); representatives for the Hampton family (Francis Andrew and myself); and representatives of the United States Justice Department (Dr. Charles Petty, a Texas medical examiner; Jerris Leonard; Jim Turner, deputy assistant attorney general; two FBI crime-detection technicians; and five U.S. marshals).

Seated at the head of a long table in the boardroom of the veterans hospital, Leonard outlined the planned procedure. Because of the small size of the dissecting room, only Dr. Petty, myself, Dr. Kearns, and Dr. Mavrelis would be permitted on the autopsy-room floor. Everyone else would sit in the observation stand nearby. Leonard also hoped that it would be possible for the pathologists representing the different factions and Dr. Petty to reach clear agreement on the currently disputed findings. If this was possible, Leonard said, the written record of this autopsy could be presented to the federal grand jury as definitive and final, eliminating the need for any of us to appear personally as witnesses.

At 4:30 P.M. we were to assemble in the morgue room across the hall from the autopsy room, where we could all witness the opening of the casket. Leonard explained that as soon as the coffin had been removed from its burial site, it had been sealed with metal strips and was thus officially certified by a U.S. marshal. This was done to prevent any later charge by any of the parties involved that the body might have been tampered with in order to alter any of the wounds.

Leonard then outlined the autopsy procedure. "After the seals are broken and the body is identified as that of Fred Hampton, it will be photographed and then removed from the casket. Following this, it will be placed on a carrier, X-rayed, further photographed, and paraffin tests will be made of the hands, fingers, and chest. When this is complete, the corpse will be taken to the dissecting room and the autopsy will begin. If the pathologists so desire, they will be given a change of clothing, aprons, and gloves in order to facilitate their participation in this examination along with Dr. Petty. Any materials or tissues taken from the body for chemical or microscopic analysis will be divided into three equal and representative portions and divided among Dr. Spain, the Illinois and Cook County pathologists, and Dr. Petty. Official copies of the final autopsy report when completed will be sent to Mr. Andrew, representing Mrs. Hampton, and the attorneys representing Cook County and the State of Illinois." Then Leonard closed the briefing session.

On my way down to the morgue, I met Dr. Petty. He mentioned that he was pleased to see me, since he had only recently had an opportunity to read a medical textbook written by me on the complications of modern medical practices—doctor-induced diseases. Dr. Petty's remarks relieved the atmosphere, which up to then had been somewhat strained. This was a far cry from the ambience of Mississippi in 1964, where I had felt like an underground agent, sneaking in and out of Jackson to get a view of the slain civil-rights workers' bodies.

Promptly at 4:30 P.M. we gathered in the morgue around the sealed casket. It was made of mahogany-colored wood, but was now soiled with dirt and partially covered with patches of greenish mold. Three broad metal bands encircled it. After the coffin was photographed to record the fact that the seals were intact, one of the United States marshals broke the seals open. Dr. Petty, assisted by me and the morgue attendant, lifted the lid off the casket.

Despite previous exposure to a number of exhumations, I was deeply moved by the sight of Hampton in his coffin. A terse description of this dramatic and startling sight was contained in the final autopsy report: "The body is partially covered by a multitude of rings and buttons and other mementos. The body is clothed in a dark-colored suit, a blue high-neck shirt with cuff-links, black shoes and socks. . . . The state of preservation of the body is excellent. . . . There is a small mustache present. The sideburns are long and extend to the level of the mouth on either side. A short and rather sparsely populated goatee is present. . . . The only scar of significance noted is one that extends from the junction of the middle of the right eyebrow. . . ."

The rings covering the body were of varied design, undoubtedly placed or dropped into the coffin as an act of respect and devotion by his brother and sister Panthers, friends, and relatives. The many buttons of varied size and color covered most of his jacket and shirt, and bore almost every known political slogan on the themes of poverty, racism, and war (and of course among these were the usual vituperative anti-police, "pig" epithets). Hampton's face appeared strangely alive, and he was strikingly handsome. He seemed very much the African tribal prince.

Jerris Leonard broke these reflections when he asked if anyone present was personally acquainted with Hampton and could officially identify the body. No one had any serious doubts about the identification, but, to my dismay, Thomas Hett, Illinois assistant state's attorney, insisted on further positive identification with fingerprints. An attempt was made to accommodate him, but the usual rigidity and the position of the fingers of the corpse made it difficult to obtain satisfactory prints. Hett then suggested that the fingers be cut off so that they could be rolled individually on the ink pad. It is to Jerris Leonard's credit that he balked at this request; he did not see any reason for this needless mutilation of the body. Hett was persuaded to desist. He never had really doubted that the body was really that of Fred Hampton, but for some reason he suddenly became a stickler for meticulous legal procedure and detail. After all, it was his office that had been engaged in the initial, allegedly slipshod and perfunctory investigation following the raid.

To determine whether any gunpowder granules were embedded in the skin of the hands or chest, the FBI technician brushed melted paraffin over these areas. When a gun is shot, the firing pin strikes the percussion cap, at the center of the base of the cartridge, and the impact detonates the primer. This in turn ignites the powder or propellent charge, and the large amount of gas that is evoked forces the pellet on its way. Simultaneously the gas may backfire, scattering powder granules onto the skin of the person firing the weapon, especially if the weapon is somewhat faulty. When powder granules are embedded in the skin, they are picked up by the paraffin, which can then be examined. The presence of powder granules is suggestive evidence that the individual may have recently fired a gun. The failure to find powder granules does not conclusively prove that a gun has not been fired by the individual in question, but, with other, supporting evidence, it may lead us to think that there hasn't been gunplay. When the paraffin used in this autopsy hardened, the casts were removed and placed in sepa-

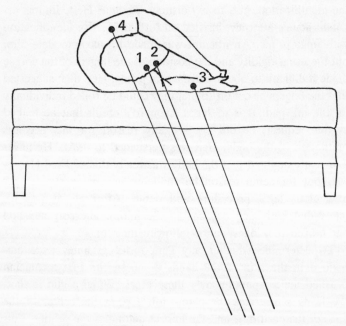

Entries of the four bullets.

rate labeled envelopes indicating the parts from which they had been obtained.

The preliminary procedures seemed to drag on at a snail's pace. It was now almost 6:00 P.M. I had previously arranged to be picked up by Mrs. Hampton and taken to the airport at 8:30 P.M. There was only one plane out that evening for New York, and it was essential that I be back the next morning, since I had a previous commitment to chair an important meeting. I had anticipated that with the autopsy scheduled to begin at 4:30 P.M., I would have ample time to make my plane. I was now beginning to doubt this. Dr. Petty was proceeding very slowly, making the most minute preliminary observations, almost all of which were irrelevant to the main issues of the case. However, it must be said that he was thorough; he probably did not want to be accused at a later date of any particular oversight. The organs that had been dissected at the previous autopsies were found in a plastic bag within the abdomen. This was opened, the organs were examined, and portions of the liver were given to each of the participants for their own, further chemical analysis. Finally, at 6:00 P.M., the body was moved into the autopsy room and the re-examination of the significant wounds begun.

The crucial moment in the autopsy had been reached. Dr. Petty had now begun to study the disputed wound in the forehead. It had been diagnosed as an exit wound by the Cook County coroner's pathologist and as an entry wound by the Panthers' pathologist, Dr. Victor Levine. While Dr. Petty was examining this area and before he openly announced his opinion, it was evident to me that the skull wound fulfilled all the criteria of an entry bullet-hole wound and thus confirmed Dr. Victor Levine's finding.

When a bullet enters bone, it bores a hole that widens out. The exit side of the bone is beveled due to the widening of the disintegrating force of the bullet as it spreads out in the bone. In the case of a skull wound, on the entry side the outer table of bone is not broken up, but the inner table is. In an exit wound through the skull, the reverse is true, with widening of the beveled zone on the outer surface of the outer table, which has been broken away as the bullet leaves the skull.

So it came as no surprise when Dr. Petty said the forehead injury was an entry wound. Suddenly, at this point, Dr. Kearns and Dr. Mavrelis strenuously objected to Petty's conclusion. This only succeeded in irritating him, because their disagreement was not supported by any scientific evidence. The exit component and the track leading from this entry wound were located on the left side of the face in front of the ear; it had been obscured by the hair of the sideburns. This was the wound that Dr. Levine had not seen. This oversight was of little import to the proper interpretation of the trajectory of the bullet, because this was already clearly delineated by the other wounds and by the entry component and interior track of this wound.

There was more embarrassment to the representatives from Illinois when no entry wound was found in the right side of the neck, as they had so plainly described. This bullet hole was actually in front of the right ear, over the cheekbone, as reported by Dr. Levine. The shoulder wound and the superficial wound over the right forearm were found as originally described.

One other observation proved to be significant. This was the fact that the stomach as found at this autopsy was intact; there was no incision in it and there was no evidence that it had ever been opened or examined. The importance of this became evident in relation to the sworn testimony of the Cook County pathologist before the grand jury that he had opened the stomach.

It was now about 8:30 P.M., and as far as I was concerned, the crucial portion of the autopsy had been completed. I therefore thanked Dr. Petty and Mr. Leonard for the courtesy extended to me and departed. Once outside the hospital, I was picked up by Mrs. Hampton and her sister and driven to the airport. I later learned that Dr. Petty had continued along with his slow, methodical, detailed procedure and actually had not finished the autopsy until well after midnight.

On my flight back I realized that a half-smoked and partially chewed cigar had never left Dr. Petty's mouth. He'd never stopped puffing away during his entire autopsy dissection. As a matter of fact, that aspect of his behavior had rather disconcerted me. Years back, when I was a young assistant pathologist in training, I was imbued with the importance of a dignified and respectful atmosphere in the autopsy room by my boss, the elderly Dr. Symmers. Every so often he would come into the large autopsy room in the old Bellevue Hospital. With a slow, stiff, somewhat unsteady gait he would approach anyone who might be smoking and snatch the cigarette from the startled individual's mouth. "No smoking in the presence of death." Professor Symmers would then make a sharp about-face and stalk slowly from the room.

After my return to New York, I learned that chemical analysis of the tissue taken at this third and final autopsy failed to show the presence of any sleep-inducing drugs in Hampton's body.

For the next two months there were no new developments, and there existed a self-imposed silence by all parties concerned, who were awaiting the release of the conclusions of the 1970 federal grand jury report. On May 15, 1970, the results of their deliberations were made public and revealed that no indictment had been handed down. According to the New York *Times* that day, "the issuance of a narrative report rather than indictments by a Federal Grand Jury is extremely unusual." Although there were no indictments, one positive result issued from the report: all charges of attempted murder (for which the seven

Panthers who survived the raid had been indicted) were dismissed. And three high-ranking Chicago police officials were demoted. This led a lawyer for the American Civil Liberties Union to charge at a news conference that he believed that a "deal" had been made: in exchange for the police dropping the attempted murder charges against the Panthers, the grand jury had declined to return any indictments against the police.

A careful reading of the full report listed many telling irregularities on the part of the Chicago police and the local official investigating agencies. For example, four officers testified that they had seen a female Panther fire a shot from a shotgun at them. The grand jury concluded, on the basis of the relative positions of the woman and the police, that this was a physical impossibility. Eight officers testified they had heard or seen shots originating from the north bedroom. But only one shotgun was found in that room, and none of the expended shells recovered either in that room or elsewhere in the apartment had been fired from that gun. The grand jury was moved to ask whether the officers were falsifying their accounts. Nevertheless the police were absolved of any premeditated wrongdoing and of violation of any individual's civil rights. The conclusions were vague and failed to come to grips with the central issues of the case.

It was a surprise to read in the grand jury report the following: "Fortunately, the misdescription of the right head wound as a wound of exit does not seem to have substantive effect on this case." Nothing could be farther from the truth. The final and correct placement of these wounds was conclusive and critical to a proper interpretation of this case, because it proved that Fred Hampton was shot in full view of his killer and in a defenseless position—not in a blind shoot-out.

Taking into consideration the location of the bed in the south bedroom of the raided apartment, the position of the door leading to this bedroom, and the angle of entrance of the bullet holes through the walls and their projected trajectory, the most plausible position of Fred Hampton's body at the time of the shooting that could adequately account for the location and direction of bullet wounds in his body was that he was lying on his right side with his head turned toward the right and his right arm positioned under his head, with his face toward the south wall. This is the only position that most logically accounts for all the entry wounds and their trajectories, especially the entry wound over the right cheekbone and its exit from the left side of the throat, and the forehead entry with its exit through the left sideburn. These two wounds line up with the wound in the left shoulder and the grazed right forearm. All the bullets could only have come from the direction of the open door leading into the south bedroom. No other position of the body and no other origin and direction of the shots, no matter how one twists and turns, can satisfactorily put all the proven facts into one uniform, logical picture.

It is interesting to note that the bullet removed from Fred Hampton's chest muscle was assumed, in the federal grand jury report, to have come through the bedroom wall. No matter how one positions the body of Fred Hampton on the bed, this was clearly not possible. In the first place it was proved that the only bullets that came through the wall were at shoulder height and couldn't have hit anyone on the bed. Secondly, if Hampton had been lying on his stomach, as the police reported, his right shoulder would have been placed to the wall, and the direction of the wound would have been toward the outer side of his body, not, as was the case, in the opposite direction. Was this casually stated and farfetched assumption innocently, accidentally, or deliberately recorded in the federal grand jury report?

And somewhat disconcerting was the failure to include the results of the paraffin test. One must assume, therefore, that no powder granules were found on Hampton's fingers, hands, or chest.

At the final autopsy, and mentioned in the grand jury report, was the observation that the stomach was found to be intact and had never been opened. In this same grand jury report it is noted that the Chicago coroner's pathologist had testified under oath that he had opened the stomach and found its contents to be fluid. It is surprising in view of all these clear and unequivocal facts that the grand jury did not hand down any indictments for perjury or violation of civil rights—or for murder.

The New York *Times* felt there was sufficient hard evidence disclosed in the report to publish a lead editorial on May 19, 1970, that stated, in part: "The unusual narrative by the Federal Grand Jury in the Chicago police raid which killed two Black Panthers last December confirms earlier suspicions of a police shoot-in rather than a Panther shoot-out. The evidence adds up to a flagrant case of police violence, followed by official distortion. Moreover, the Chicago police appeared to have taken the offensive with the advice and consent of the Federal Bureau of Investigation. . . . Against a background of doctored evidence and coached police witnesses, it is not surprising that the State's Attorney, who had initially played a leading role in building a public case against the Panthers, finally dropped all charges against them. A more pertinent question now is whether a case which left two men dead can properly be closed with the mere demotion of three police officials."

The grand jury placed the blame for their failure to take any further action on the Panthers' refusal to co-operate with them by testifying at the hearings.

A New York *Times* editorial chastised the Panthers for the same reason. In response to this, I sent a letter to the *Times*. After several weeks of negotiation concerning their request to delete certain statements, the letter was finally published, on

June 6, 1970. In it, I briefly outlined the two errors or "distortions" uncovered by the second autopsy, in order to indicate that the Panthers' version of the incident was substantially correct. I said that I had seen several cases of either distorted or dishonest conclusions derived from official autopsies, despite the fact that the autopsy is supposed to be non-political and scientifically objective. I continued, "My experience and the recent events in Chicago tend to support the attitude of the Chicago Panthers who refused to participate in the recent investigation, saying that they could only trust their peers. They seem to have good reason for this.

"The blame for incompetent or distorted autopsy reports cannot be placed entirely upon the politically motivated coroner's office, but can also occur even in politically independent medical examiners' offices when there is a lack of individual integrity and a scientifically sound approach to any examination."

Of particular personal interest was the federal grand jury's remarks as to the competence and performance of the Chicago coroner's office. For twenty years I have advocated replacing the antiquated coroner system with modern medical examiners' departments staffed by well-trained pathologists. This would place all the investigative and inquest functions in the district attorney's office and leave the strictly medical aspects to the specialists in forensic medicine. I have spoken on this subject at many county and state medical societies. The grand jury agreed. It concluded, "The office of the Coroner [referring to Illinois], as in other states, is a combination of archaic and statutory functions. This investigation establishes reasonable grounds to question whether the continuation of that office is desirable. . . . Nor did the medical work of the coroner's office seem to be of high calibre. The reversal of the entrance and the exit holes and the misdescription of one of the Hampton

wounds could, in some cases, have caused serious repercussions."

Until this case, I had held the mistaken impression that the
Chicago coroner's system was staffed by competent forensic
pathologists. As the Hampton case unfolded, I soon realized
that the Illinois system was no different from those states described by the National Municipal League, where, in their words,
"one commits murder with relative safety." There are still too
many communities where deaths unattended by physicians are
investigated by a typical county coroner, a lay politico elected
on the tail end of a political-party ticket, who knows nothing
of pathology, let alone pathology's capacity to make dead men
tell tales.

I busied myself with a written analysis of the conflicting autopsy reports on behalf of the commission of inquiry, feeling
more sanguine about the value of this report.

Toward the end of 1971, when the commission of inquiry
was putting the finishing touches to its report, Ramsay Clark,
the former attorney general, asked me to meet with him to iron
out an unsettled question about the position of Hampton's body
at the time of death.

Anyone coming upon the scene in Ramsay Clark's office
would have been perplexed. This tall, thin, and gracious man
was stretched out on the couch and I was bent over him, manip-
ulating his head into different positions and making certain
measurements. A few minutes later our positions were reversed
and he was moving my head—all for the purpose of resolving
some of his doubts concerning the Hampton case. At the end
we arrived at substantial agreement.

I have always been intrigued by individuals like Ramsay
Clark, who as attorney general in President Johnson's cabinet
could preside at the federal indictment of the noted Dr. Benjamin Spock on the charge of conspiracy for his anti-war activi-

ties, and later, as a private citizen, officiate at the awarding of an honor to Dr. Spock for the very same "crimes." It is ironic that he has recently contributed to the legal defense of Father Berrigan, similarly indicted by his old employer, the Justice Department—for alleged conspiratorial peace activities. I know, though, that thoughtful men can change their minds: as medical examiner of Westchester County, I used to work alongside the county district attorney. After I resigned, I worked the other side of the street as the expert witness for the defense against these same prosecuting district attorneys.

In the anteroom to Clark's office, Leonard Boudin, an old friend and perhaps the leading legal authority on constitutional questions affecting civil liberties, stopped to chat with me. His brilliant advocacy in First Amendment cases had led to a number of Supreme Court landmark decisions. He had been working with Clark on the Berrigan brothers' defense. (Most recently, he participated in Daniel Ellsberg's defense in the Pentagon Papers trial.) He expressed a general sense of futility and purposelessness despite his many successes in civil liberties. Thinking about his remarks at a later date, I felt that Boudin's feeling of despair stems from his isolating his work on these constitutional questions from the totality of the human struggle for betterment. In a sense, he was treating civil liberties as an end in itself—a sort of art for art's sake approach. I have only rarely experienced this sense of hopelessness, I believe, because I have never separated civil-rights pathology from the remainder of the struggle.

During this time, internecine warfare erupted within the ranks of the Panthers. Eldridge Cleaver, Panther minister of information and later a refugee in Algiers, was expelled from the organization by Huey Newton. Cleaver in turn threatened Newton's expulsion. Michael Tabor and Richard Moore, local New York Panther leaders on trial in New York, jumped $150,000

bail and were allegedly said to be in Algiers; they were also
read out of the party by Newton. The Oakland-based Panthers
accused Cleaver of holding Kathleen, his wife, a virtual prisoner.
The New York Panthers accused the West Coast group of send-
ing "mad dog assassins" to kill New York Panther Robert
Webb, a local deputy field marshal. Webb was found dead, and
the case is still under investigation. Edward Jay Epstein, writing
in *The New Yorker* magazine, challenged the prevalent assumption that twenty-four Panthers had been deliberately killed by
the police. To make matters worse, the threats and counter-
threats, expulsions and counterexpulsions, and the scandalous
charges and countercharges—all carried out in public—have
pretty much canceled out the credibility of any serious political
dispute. Panther defendants currently on trial justly or unjustly
now can be sure of receiving harsher "justice" than heretofore.

Because of the Panthers' sudden unattractiveness to so many
former well-wishers, I wasn't surprised when some of my friends
asked me to justify my continued involvement on behalf of Mrs.
Hampton, particularly in the presence of such a "disagreeable
and disgusting spectacle." These friends have missed the point.
My reason for staying with this case had nothing to do with
politics or ideology. I wanted to get at the truth—to discover
whether a man's civil rights and civil liberties had been violated.
My involvement is concerned entirely with the elemental human
rights, the dignity of any single individual regardless of the circumstances. Each potential assault on anyone's basic human
rights must be relentlessly explored, whether that person be an
alleged murderer, an alleged traitor, an alleged radical, an alleged terrorist, an alleged rapist, or anyone else categorized as
being beyond the pale. Otherwise, the entire premise of our Bill
of Rights, and the legal procedures for safeguarding these rights,
becomes no more nor less than an intellectual and judicial fraud.
My *raison d'être* is what Jacques Barzun, Columbia University

provost, considers a traditional American right: "pursuit of one's idea or defense of the truth, regardless of respectability." Also one must realize that the Panthers are desperate men—their desperation growing out of frustration, helplessness and degradation —and so they engage in desperate acts.

The pursuit of truth in this case has not yet ended. On April 26, 1971, stories broke in the national press about widespread reports in Chicago that a special Cook County grand jury had voted indictments against Cook County State's Attorney Edward V. Hanrahan and other law-enforcement officials connected with the raid on the Panthers' apartment.

For a few months the release of this indictment was blocked by the maneuvers of Mayor Daley's political machine. In the fall of 1971 an indictment of Hanrahan on the charges of obstructing the pursuit of justice in the raid on the Panthers became official and was finally made public. Eventually Hanrahan was found not guilty.

Perhaps the Fred Hampton *cause célèbre* is not over. Why the stubborn pursuit? A principle has been at stake. Although the injustice already done could not be remedied, at least it could have been admitted. The Hampton affair was a glaring way station on the road to the current wave of morally and politically indefensible (and self-defeating) ambush assassinations of police. It was neither the beginning nor the end. Arising out of growing frustration, failure, and desperation, it was a prelude to one black militant's prophecy of the coming "shitstorm"—the accelerated social disintegration caused by the disparate factions on the American scene.

4. DEATH IN THE TOMBS—THE CASE OF RAYMOND LAVON MOORE

It destroys the logical processes of the mind, a man's thoughts become completely disorganized. The noise, madness screaming from every throat, frustrated sounds from the bars, metallic sounds from the walls, the steel trays, the iron beds bolted to the wall, the hollow sounds from a cast-iron sink or toilet. . . . The smells of human waste thrown at us, unwashed bodies, the rotten food. . . .

George Jackson, in a letter from Soledad Prison

When Raymond Lavon Moore was found hanging in his cell in New York's men's house of detention (the Tombs) on November 3, 1970, the official autopsy report showed a verdict of death by suicide. It was the seventh suicide in the New York City jails during the year, and this alarming figure galvanized both the city's Department of Corrections and the watchdog Board of Corrections headed by Chairman William J. vanden Heuvel.

The department's knee-jerk reaction was to issue a statement that, just two days before, Moore had attacked a guard and broken his nose. The report went on to state that Moore had hanged himself on November 3, using a rope formed of mattress ticking. The department said that it had been "trying for months to get him committed" to Bellevue Hospital and that he had made two earlier attempts at suicide.

Moore's father wanted a new autopsy; his suspicions had been aroused by the funeral director in Newburgh, New York—his home town—who had received the embalmed body of Raymond Moore. The funeral director thought there was evidence of injuries not mentioned in the city medical examiner's report. Ned Kopald, the elder Moore's lawyer, called me on November 7 and asked me if I would agree to reautopsy Raymond Moore's body. I said I would.

By this time, Vanden Heuvel had also become involved in the case on behalf of the Board of Corrections. He and I had worked together once before in the investigation of another Tombs suicide—that of Julio Roldan, a Puerto Rican and member of the Young Lords, a militant Puerto Rican group. Roldan had been charged with setting a street fire in a neighborhood garbage protest. The Lords, suspicious of the manner of Roldan's death, had retained me as an independent expert to make a report of the case, which the medical examiner's office had declared a suicide. I stood by on their behalf while the medical examiner performed the autopsy. The autopsy revealed no evidence of any beating, and the findings supported the original conclusion that Roldan's death had been suicide by hanging. I reported to the Lords that I concurred with the medical examiner in the finding of suicide.

Vanden Heuvel felt that my conclusions in the Roldan case demonstrated both to him and the public my objectivity and credibility as an independent observer. He requested that I keep him informed of the results of my examination.

My first step was to contact Dr. Michael M. Baden, acting deputy chief medical examiner, who had performed the first autopsy and reached a verdict of suicide by hanging. He had found no evidence of beating. When I finally reached him, I asked him to fill me in on his findings. He described an injury to the left side of the head, with an attendant skull fracture, but added that these injuries had undoubtedly occurred after the suicide victim's death, when the body hit the cell floor after being cut down. I asked him if he had taken any pieces of tissue from the site of the head injury for microscopic study (this is the only sure method of determining whether the head injury has occurred during life). Dr. Baden replied without hesitation that he had indeed taken a tissue sample.

I wondered whether Dr. Baden might have overlooked taking tissue specifically from the scalp wounds at the original autopsy, and on the basis of incomplete evidence had prejudged the timing of the head injury. My doubts remained when I subsequently read a copy of his official autopsy report; no mention was made of the taking of such sections, nor was there a description of them. Dr. Baden had reached and disclosed his conclusions without waiting for the results of any tissue examination.

Dr. Baden's official autopsy report listed only the following injuries and pertinent observations:

"Circumferential abrasion about the neck [caused by the noose of mattress stripping];

Crusted lacerations [cuts] on the front of the wrists;

Fresh and old scars on the front of the left wrist;

Recently ingested food in the stomach—undigested, intact rice granules and green bean fragments [no digested or partially digested food particles were noted in the intestinal continuation from the stomach];

Fracture of skull—*fresh;*

Ecchymosis [hemorrhage], left scalp [overlying the fracture area];

Half-inch long *abrasion* above the left eyebrow." (Emphasis mine.)

Dr. Milton Helpern, chief medical examiner, called that evening. He was friendly and thanked me for the courtesy of informing his office of the contemplated re-examination. As an aside, he mentioned how unfortunate it was that so few of those retained to reautopsy cases originating from his office had the same good manners. He said the district attorney would like someone from his office to be present at my examination. This was perfectly acceptable to me, and I told him the autopsy would be done at 8:00 A.M. the next day, at Doulan's Funeral Home, in Newburgh. I cautioned him that whomever he sent as an observer had to be on time, because, firstly, the funeral was scheduled for later that same morning and, secondly, only I had permission to autopsy the body and take tissue from it at this time.

Promptly at 8:00 A.M., the re-examination of the body of Raymond Lavon Moore was begun. Assembled at Doulan's Funeral Parlor to witness the procedure were Ned Kopald, a local embalmer, and a Newburgh police detective who also served as photographer. Missing was the representative from the New York medical examiner's office.

The second autopsy uncovered a number of injuries not previously described in Dr. Baden's official report. There were two additional distinct and separate head wounds, an area of extensive hemorrhage covering the back of the right hand, and a deep hemorrhagic contusion over the right shinbone. Dr. Baden's appraisal of the wound over the left eyebrow had been miserably understated. Instead of a superficial abrasion, it was a deep and gaping wound reaching to the surface of the skull bone. Also, the injury over the left side of the head was twice as big as originally described.

All the injuries were photographed, and bits of tissue were removed from the wound sites for subsequent microscopic study to determine if the injuries had occurred during life and, if so, approximately how long before death.

The examination was completed at 9:30 A.M. By this time we were certain no one from New York was going to show. We left, and in a nearby diner over a cup of coffee, Kopald filled me in on some of the background of this case. The deceased had been jailed in the Tombs for eight months awaiting trial, because the extremely high bail, set at fifteen thousand dollars, could not be raised. Moore had been charged with attempted assault in a barroom argument, during which a gun had discharged accidentally, injuring an off-duty patrolman who was sitting nearby. Moore had had no previous criminal record. Mr. Kopald suspected that he had been beaten by the prison guards (probably, I thought, because he had allegedly wounded an officer) and that perhaps his death was really not due to suicide. Tragically, a few days before his demise, bail had been reduced, and he was to have been released. I suggested we suspend any further discussion or speculation until I had time to study the tissue sections and could definitely determine when the injuries had been inflicted.

Upon returning to my laboratory at Brookdale Hospital, I found a message from the mortician; Dr. Baden had arrived at the funeral home late, a few minutes after our departure, and had taken pieces of tissue from the self-inflicted lacerations of the wrists.

I asked my technicians to rush the preparation of the tissue sections. Twenty-four hours later, the slides were ready, and microscopic examination of them proved unequivocally that Raymond Moore had sustained the soft-tissue injuries of the scalp, eyebrow, hand, and leg while still alive. It is an established elementary biologic fact that the human body responds to noxious intruders, including trauma (a blow or gash), by mobilizing thousands of small sentinels (white blood cells, leucocytes) at the injured part of the body. This is a vital reaction; it can occur only in a living animal. We call this reaction *inflammation.* There are several basic types of these cells, and they arrive at the wound in a regular sequence, which takes from about two to forty-eight hours. In addition, repair cells become visible about twenty-four hours after the injury has been sustained, and these scar-tissue cells, along with the leucocytes, are easily spotted through the microscope. In the specimens of injured tissue from Moore's body, the number and types of cells seen established an approximate time when the injuries were likely to have occurred. These tissue studies proved conclusively that the wounds had been inflicted while the victim was still alive, probably about forty-eight hours before death. Here the facts were clear and unmistakable.

There were other items recorded in Dr. Baden's report that needed clarification and raised disturbing questions. One of these was the presence in the stomach of undigested rice granules and beans. Another was the absence of the small hemorrhages frequently and characteristically seen in the eyelids, scalp, and neck region in strangulation deaths caused by hanging (the lack of oxygen and the pressure on the neck forces the blood to seep through the walls of the blood vessels).

With Mr. Kopald's consent, these observations were reported to Mr. Vanden Heuvel, but not before evaluating the extent to which we thought he would go in pursuit of the complete story. Kopald and I sensed that Vanden Heuvel was basically decent, humane, and well meaning, but we also were aware that he was politically ambitious, with his sights possibly set on the governorship of the state. Under these circumstances, would he risk antagonizing key individuals in his party and go all the way with us, or would he balk at the first sign of trouble and expediently withdraw to avoid conflict, or compromise the issue? We decided to be completely open with him, and never regretted our decision.

A few days later, Ned Kopald and I met with him and showed

him the photographs, the results of the microscopic examination, and my completed autopsy report. We discussed the difference between my observations and conclusions and those of the city medical examiner.

We concluded that at least five injuries had been inflicted on the deceased during his life and in all likelihood had been sustained during a beating or an altercation; that some of the head injuries could have been caused by a blunt weapon; that the injuries in and of themselves, though not necessarily lethal, could nevertheless have caused considerable pain and suffering —enough to aggravate a suicidal impulse in a person with the temperament, troubles, and frustrations of Raymond Moore.

The undigested food particles in the stomach were not consistent with a guard's claim that Moore was last seen alive at 10:30 P.M.; he was known to have eaten at 6:30 P.M., and four hours is more than sufficient for the stomach to be emptied of most of its food content. At the least, the stomach should have contained partially or almost completely digested material; it should certainly not contain food in the condition described in Baden's report.

If Moore was actually dead at 10:30 P.M., why was this falsified? What was actually going on in the vicinity of Moore's "punishment" cell in the few hours prior to the time he was reported dead? Was it technically feasible for Moore to have hanged himself under the conditions existing in a tight-security cell? We speculated whether he had been strung up by the guards in order to conceal that he had been beaten or had died from a beating.

Mr. Vanden Heuvel was satisfied with the reliability of our data. He now revealed an episode heretofore unknown to us, an event that had led him to suspect there was more to Moore's death than showed on the surface. On Sunday evening, November 1, as Chairman of the Board of Corrections, he made a

surprise inspection tour of the Tombs and inadvertently crossed
paths with one of the prison guards, who rushed past him, hands
covering his face and bleeding from the nose. Naturally Vanden
Heuvel's curiosity was aroused and he questioned the guard,
who explained he had been attacked by one of the inmates.
He claimed that prisoner Raymond Moore had been screaming
and complaining about a mistake in the medication given to
him. Responding to this disturbance, he had rushed to Moore's
cell and, as he'd approached the cell door, Moore had surprised
him by striking his nose with a shoe thrust through the space
between the bars on the cell door. The guard stated he had
not entered the cell (a strictly enforced regulation prohibits any
guard from entering an inmate's cell alone). Continuing his investigation, Vanden Heuvel next spoke to Moore, who flatly
denied the guard's story. The prisoner insisted the guard had
ordered the cell door "broken" (prison lingo for getting the
door open; in the Tombs this is accomplished by an officer at
a remote-control panel). The guard then rushed at Moore, who
struck the officer with a shoe in self-defense. While talking to
Moore, Vanden Heuvel saw signs that the prisoner had recently
been beaten; Moore's shirt was bloody, and a fresh, untreated
gash extended above his left eyebrow. The guard, in turn, flatly
denied Moore's story.

In checking out the event, Vanden Heuvel tried to re-enact
the guard's version; with the shoe in his hand, he attempted
to strike out through the space between the bars. This proved
impossible; the shoe did not fit between the bars. He now
doubted the accuracy of the guard's statement. Mr. Vanden
Heuvel was especially intrigued by my statement that Moore's
injuries were probably sustained approximately forty-eight hours
prior to his death. This coincided almost exactly with Vanden
Heuvel's independent guess as to the time of the suspected assault on Moore.

Vanden Heuvel then disclosed an alleged eyewitness account of the thrashing in the form of a letter signed by several prisoners. It had been sent to him by the Young Lords. This letter, smuggled out of the Tombs to the Young Lords, told of seeing five guards, two with blackjacks, enter Moore's cell and beat him. The document named the guards and listed their badge numbers for further identification. Mr. Vanden Heuvel had gone to the Tombs, inspected the area of the alleged crime, and questioned the signees of the letter to establish the authenticity of the document and the validity of their statements. He was personally satisfied that the prisoners had been in a position to see what they had described. They showed Vanden Heuvel several small hand mirrors usually concealed on their persons; placing these at certain angles reflected a clear view of the entire area.

We were permitted to see the original copy of the letter. This fascinating penciled document, in addition to its revelation about the Moore affair, pledged political support and encouragement to the black, Puerto Rican, and "third world" brothers outside the prison walls and promised that the "liberation struggle" within the Tombs would continue.

Before setting a date for the public release of these facts, we decided it would be proper and fair to meet with Dr. Helpern in a serious and all-out effort to reconcile the differing autopsy results. The issue was not who had done a better autopsy, or who was more correct, but whether the civil rights and liberties of a prison inmate had been violated and whether any of the prison guards had committed a crime. Judicious settlement of the case could certainly be expedited if we were to reach a reasonable agreement.

Friday afternoon, we gathered in the conference room of the Forensic Medicine Institute, on First Avenue. Also present was a legal representative from Mayor Lindsay's office, and Dr.

Baden, who had hurriedly returned from a sudden vacation. Dr. Helpern made it clear at the very beginning that we were there solely at his pleasure and that he did not look upon this as a meeting of equals. He was indignant that we could question the integrity and competence of his office. Seated at the head of the long conference table, he looked every inch the autocrat. After some soft-spoken and delicately worded assurance from me that it was never our intent to challenge his department and that our sole purpose was to resolve any differences, he (on the surface at least) appeared reassured and seemed somewhat more receptive. We proceeded to the serious business at hand.

I presented the results of the second autopsy with the detailed description of the additional injuries; the photographs and the tissue preparations were used as supportive evidence. At one point, Dr. Baden challenged one of my interpretations, but Helpern, after carefully studying the microscopic sections, brushed Baden's objection aside. The facts were definitive, and without any hesitation he agreed that the soft-tissue injuries had been present before death. As a matter of fact, he blurted: "But these wounds are at least forty-eight hours old!" He seemed quite pleased with this observation, because he had apparently assumed we were about to claim they had been inflicted shortly before death and indeed were the cause of death. Concerning the skull fracture, he hedged and would not make a final judgment. He did concede the possibility that the fracture could have been there before death, but he would not allow that the blow producing the fracture was the cause of death. His argument was based on the absence of any grossly visible injury or hemorrhage in the brain. He clung to this position in the face of the printed statements and recorded experience of the country's leading brain pathologists, who have described well-documented cases of a blow to the head resulting in instantaneous death where the most meticulous examination of the brain at autopsy revealed no grossly visible sign of brain damage. I have seen this type of case, and I would bet Dr. Helpern has too.

To diminish the impact of his concession that the head and extremity injuries had occurred forty-eight hours before death, Helpern added that the wounds were "trivial." I restrained myself from saying that they might have seemed trivial to Dr. Helpern, but they hadn't been so trivial to Moore. Helpern mentioned that, since Puerto Ricans are a very excitable people, the injuries could have come from banging himself around the cell, against the bed, or against the wall. Here Vanden Heuvel interjected that the deceased was not Puerto Rican, but black. This did not seem to faze Helpern.

Dr. Baden, who hadn't said very much up to this point, was nervously jumping around from one side of the conference table to the other. He suddenly commented that the hand injury probably was caused by Moore striking out at a guard with the back of his hand. "That's possible," I said, "but also possible, and perhaps more plausible, is that the injury could have come about if Moore had held his hand in front of his face and head as protection against the guard's blows." Baden clammed up.

This short exchange between the two of us, brief as it was, highlights something that is at the very core of a pathologist's job: an honest and fair interpretation of evidence. He must give fair consideration to, and equal presentation of, all the possibilities. The physical evidence in an autopsy is incontrovertible; bias comes in when the pathologist interprets it. The only fair interpretation is one made in the context of all the evidence. There may be several different ways to explain how an injury occurred, but some explanations are obviously going to be more reasonable than others in the light of other injuries and the circumstances of death.

Thus Baden's interpretation of how the hand injury had occurred was as valid as mine; yet, with his interpretation, Moore was the aggressor; with mine, Moore was the victim. Which of us was right depended not so much on the character of the wound itself but on the context of the death injury and the other injuries.

A medical examiner must not have a hasty reaction to autopsy findings. He should present all logical explanations of the physical facts and not try to explain away an interpretation by bringing in improbable but possible interpretations of each individual injury even if the sum total of his findings do not add up to a coherent picture.

In many trials, a defendant's life is in the balance, and the jury must depend upon the neutral, intelligent, and honest interpretation of the facts by the prosecution's expert witness, the medical examiner. I believe that Baden, in an attempt to exonerate the medical examiner's office from any fault, was not treating the Moore case objectively.

Finally Vanden Heuvel asked Dr. Helpern to join with me in the formulation of a common statement spelling out the areas of agreement and disagreement. He flatly refused, and insisted on independent reports. "Let the public choose whom to believe —Dr. Helpern or Dr. Spain," he said. These abrupt remarks closed the meeting.

We had made certain gains. The medical examiner's office had now officially, if not publicly, acknowledged its original error and oversight. Without any qualification, the soft-tissue injuries except for the skull fracture had been present before death. Dr. Helpern had agreed to put this in writing. My earlier suspicion of Baden's failure to take tissue from the soft-tissue injuries of the head for microscopic study was fortified. It seemed I alone had this vital evidence.

On the way out, Ned Kopald, William vanden Heuvel, and I paused for a moment on the steps of the Forensic Medical Institute to digest the results of the meeting and to plan our next step. Ned Kopald could not resist telling us how he was amused at the change in the way Helpern and I had addressed each other as the conference progressed. In the beginning, we had been relatively informal: it had been "Milton" and "David." Later, in carefully measured tones, it had become "Doctor Helpern" and "Doctor Spain."

Vanden Heuvel was anxious to know what public stance we might expect from the medical examiner's office. To help him anticipate the nature of Helpern's response, I related the background of my more than thirty years' association with Dr. Helpern.

As a member of Bellevue's pathology staff, I had worked alongside Helpern in the hospital's gigantic autopsy room. This space was shared by the hospital's pathology department and the New York City medical examiner's office. We came to know each other quite well professionally, and during the next ten years I learned much forensic pathology from this daily contact. I have always admired Helpern's forensic skills. When I was charged with the task of establishing a new and modern medical examiner's office for Westchester County, his advice was generously offered and proved invaluable. He and I have served together as consultants on a number of reautopsies, and also in the re-examination of a few exhumed bodies. We have testified in court for the same client, and, less frequently, for opposing sides. In one of New York's most publicized murder trials, the Alice Crimmins case, he was the medical expert for the prosecution and I was the expert for the defense.

There were occasions when, for one reason or another, it was inappropriate for Helpern or a member of his staff to testify about their own findings. At these times, the interested parties called upon me to appear in their behalf to confirm the city medical examiner's findings. Many times, I have been retained by next of kin, or interested organizations such as CORE, to stand by as an observer and represent them while Helpern or some other member of his staff was doing an autopsy on a case in which there may have been a violation of the deceased's civil rights. The Moore case is the only one in this series in which my opinion was at considerable variance with the medical examiner's.

Dr. Helpern and I have both been interested in one of the nation's more catastrophic health problems, sudden death from heart attacks, and we have participated jointly on panel discussions devoted to this subject at several national medical symposia. Returning by train from one such meeting in Princeton, we got into a freewheeling discussion that gave me a great deal of insight into Helpern's personality. The Coppolino murder trial was fresh in Helpern's mind, and he was still smarting from what he seemed to regard as a personal defeat. Considering that his role was supposed to be only that of a neutral expert witness, Helpern's personal involvement seemed excessive.

Briefly, Dr. Carl Coppolino, an anesthetist, had been accused of murdering the husband of a friendly neighbor. In the first of the two Coppolino trials, Helpern was hired by the New Jersey state prosecuting attorney to testify as an expert witness. Helpern found that the victim had died from asphyxia due to the forcible prevention of air getting into the windpipe. He testified that this was an unnatural death—a homicide. F. Lee Bailey, the noted defense counsel, produced as his expert Dr. Joseph Spellman, Philadelphia's chief medical examiner, who argued that death had been a natural one, from a heart attack caused by arteriosclerosis. Dr. Helpern denied there was sufficient arteriosclerosis to have produced a heart attack. The jury in its deliberations chose to believe Dr. Spellman. Coppolino was acquitted. In the other trial, held in Florida, Coppolino was charged with the murder of his wife. Again there was the same cast of characters, F. Lee Bailey and Dr. Milton Helpern. At this time, Coppolino was judged guilty. The decisive element in this verdict was Dr. Helpern's conclusion that death was caused by an injection of succinylcholine (a drug sometimes used by anesthetists as a muscle relaxant); and yet, according to F. Lee Bailey, in *The Defense Never Rests,* Helpern had admitted that his findings weren't even solid enough for publication. Helpern, in discussing this case with me, revealed so great a feeling against Dr. Spellman that in my mind he appeared to be the judge, the prosecuting attorney, and the jury. I could see myself fearing this man. I believe he had come to regard himself as infallible.

In a more expansive mood, on the same train ride, he suddenly offered me a job in his department as deputy chief medical examiner. He said he needed a trusted aid. I never knew whether the offer was a serious one or just conversation. I never pursued it; my interest had long since shifted to the more academic and general-medical aspects of pathology.

I hoped some of the details of my association with Helpern had helped Vanden Heuvel and Kopald judge what to expect. I wanted them to understand that they could not hope for the least co-operation from him in tracking down the unsolved elements of this case. And I also suspected that the District Attorney's office would not budge without the green light from Helpern.

There was not the slightest doubt in my mind that Helpern's report to Vanden Heuvel would concede the validity of the findings in the second autopsy on Moore. But in an erudite and verbose discussion of the various alternative explanations, he would diminish their significance, thus muddying rather than clarifying the events leading to Moore's death. I was so sure that his report would befuddle the issue that I told Vanden Heuvel and Kopald we would have to go it alone.

The report, when it did arrive, proved me right. In Helpern's statement the profuse use of Talmudic counterpoint and the skillful interplay of argument and counterargument yielded nothing that would allow the lay public to reach an intelligent judgment of the case. And yet there was not a single sentence that, taken by itself, could be assailed. Classic was his use of the word "scuffle" instead of "beating," "altercation," "thrashing," or "assault" to describe what had taken place. Who ever heard of a scuffle producing four blunt-weapon-induced head wounds?

Upon receipt of the two separate statements, the Board of Corrections reviewed the circumstances of Moore's death. Then Vanden Heuvel called a press conference. My statement, which he released, contained the following observations:

1) In addition to his self-inflicted wrist cuts, Raymond Lavon Moore had sustained damage to six areas of his body. Although these injuries (except the skull fracture) were not a direct cause of death, they could have produced sufficient pain and suffering to have prompted a suicide in a person as emotionally disturbed as Moore.

2) He had not received any medical treatment for his injuries, and had the father of the deceased not requested a reautopsy, none of this information would have been uncovered. Even more disturbing was the haste with which Dr. Baden concluded that the head injury was sustained after death. Again, had there been no reautopsy, his conclusion would have been final and have stood as official fact.

3) The finding of undigested food in his stomach—and the absence of the telltale pinhead-sized areas of hemorrhage in the eyelids, scalp, and about the neck contusion, so characteristic of hanging deaths—raised certain questions and required further investigation.

In the question-and-answer period of Vanden Heuvel's television presentation of the Board of Corrections' deliberations, one reporter inquired if he supported "Dr. Spain's autopsy findings rather than those in the medical examiner's report." To my astonishment, he replied: "Dr. Spain speaks for himself." This response was such a contrast to the impression of Vanden Heuvel I had gained in private that I felt a personal hurt. For the first time, I began to doubt the firmness of his stance in any ultimate showdown.

A grand-jury investigation of the Raymond Moore case was called for, but there was no immediate response, and the case disappeared from public view.

During this period, the leaders of the Young Lords contacted me and presented evidence gathered from prison inmates that alleged that "strange events" had taken place in and around Moore's cell in the final hours of his life. The Lords thought they had sufficient proof of murder. I told them that if the alleged facts could be verified, my original and tentative conclusion of suicide would have to be rescinded. Subsequently Vanden Heuvel told me that he had been unable to authenticate any of their claims.

For another reason entirely, I had welcomed this meeting with some of the Young Lords. I had a score to settle with them. My grievance stemmed from their irresponsible distortion of the information I had given to their legal representative at the conclusion of the autopsy of Julio Roldan, whose suicide had preceded Raymond Moore's death by two weeks. I had been retained by them to observe the examination performed by Dr. Devlin, a deputy chief medical examiner. Dr. Helpern also witnessed the examination. I agreed with Dr. Devlin that there was no evidence of any beating. Death was clearly caused by asphyxia due to hanging. This was the gist of my report to the Young Lords. For some peculiar reason, they quoted me to the newspapers as having told them Roldan's body was covered with bruises from a beating.

Baffled by this misquote and concerned for my personal repu-

tation and usefulness in the civil-rights movement as well as
for the false allegation against Dr. Devlin, I immediately assured
Dr. Helpern that I had reported no such thing. If he desired,
I would make a public disclaimer. This proved unnecessary, because after a member of the Human Rights Commission contacted me and learned the truth, the case was closed. The Young
Lords made no further charges.

Now it was important to clarify this matter with the Young
Lords, and I did so at the conclusion of our discussion of the
Moore case.

I minced no words in telling them what I thought of their
dishonest report to the press. By falsifying facts, they could only
corrupt and weaken their efforts. I made it clear that if they
should wish to use my professional services again, they would
have to adhere strictly to the truth. Juan Gonzalez, their main
spokesman, admitted to me that they had had serious misgivings
about the incident themselves. They had had a group discussion
immediately afterward and had criticized themselves for it. He
assured me it would never happen again. Just before the meeting
broke up, I startled them by saying, half jokingly, "In the future
we will deal with each other on a day-to-day basis of mutual
mistrust."

In the interim, I also learned from Mr. Vanden Heuvel that
someone in the city medical examiner's office had sent one or
more letters to various reporters on the New York newspapers
stating that my qualifications and experience as a pathologist
were inadequate to make any valid determinations in cases of
this sort. Levinson of CBS and Jean Crafton of the *Daily News*
informed me of other wild accusations, said to be coming from
an individual or individuals in the medical examiner's office,
to the effect that I was "unreliable, a liar, and incompetent."
These guerrilla attacks on my ability and character reached the
stage where Ned Kopald suggested legal action against the cul-

prits. I rejected this approach. I have learned from previous situations never to become personally embroiled in, or respond to, such charges. Sooner or later the real facts will out. In this instance, the truth came faster than expected, and from an unexpected source.

On January 11, 1971, the three major New York newspapers carried headlines to the effect that four prison guards had been suspended in the death of Raymond Moore (a fifth had already left for reasons of "health"). Arthur Blake, a prison guard, had finally made a statement to the *Daily News,* and then to Chairman Vanden Heuvel, that he had been a witness to the beating of Raymond Moore. According to Blake, after one guard was already in Moore's cell, four more guards rushed into the cell, two allegedly carrying blackjacks. The first guard held Moore, while the other guards beat the prisoner until he crumpled to the floor. The prisoner crawled out of the cell, his face and head bleeding. He was then handcuffed, denied medical treatment, and placed in solitary confinement and kept there until his body was found hanging from the bars of a cell window. With this revelation, District Attorney Frank Hogan called the grand jury into session to investigate the case of Raymond Lavon Moore.

On the evening before my grand-jury appearance, a longstanding friend—a medical examiner in another county—warned me, "They're out to do a job on you." Someone from the New York district attorney's office had checked with him to uncover any glaring deficiencies that might exist in my credentials. In the course of their conversation, the district attorney's man had implied that the main objective of the hearing was to restore the public's confidence in Helpern's office. Getting at all the facts in Moore's death was only a secondary concern. I was tipped off to prepare for a series of hostile questions.

On February 2, 1971, I appeared before the grand jury to

present testimony on the injuries and circumstances of the death of Raymond Moore. I was on the witness stand for two hours. I was conscious of such hostility toward me on the part of the assistant district attorney that I wasn't quite sure whether or not I was actually a defendant of some kind. He seemed to have an overriding concern with protecting the image of the medical examiner's office. All the corny tricks were used. This was patently obvious to me but completely escaped the grand jury. The assistant district attorney asked if I was paid for my work in this case. My answer was, "Yes." This is an often-used question that has no bearing on the central issues of the case. It is similar to that cliché "And when did you stop beating your wife?" In answering this, you're damned if you do and damned if you don't. If you answer yes you're being paid, your questioner intimates you are doing it for the money (everyone knows some people will sell their souls for money). If you answer no, he intimates you have such an overriding personal interest in the outcome that you cannot give fair testimony. The assistant district attorney attempted to prove I was Vanden Heuvel's man, "in his pocket," and that he had hired me for this job.

The cleverest maneuver was to sandwich my testimony between Baden's and Helpern's. This gave the appearance of two minor figures, Baden and me, having a dispute that the impartial third party—Helpern—would resolve. The separate issues of the earlier injuries and the final cause of death were deliberately merged and confused. I sometimes wonder in amazement, considering the final outcome of the grand jury's deliberations, that I was not indicted on some Kafkaesque charge.

The grand jury concluded there was no evidence of any criminal acts or any malfeasance of duties by any of the prison officials or guards. All were completely exonerated, and the matter, as far as the grand jury and the district attorney's office were concerned, was closed.

Then, on February 16, four United States congressmen signed a letter to U. S. Attorney Whitney North Seymour, Jr., asking to reopen the investigation of Raymond Moore's death. They wondered whether the New York grand jury "may be white-washing this matter and possibly sweeping the facts under the rug." The letter was signed by Representatives Edward I. Koch and Bella Abzug, both of Manhattan, Representative Benjamin S. Rosenthal of Queens, and Representative John G. Dow, from Moore's home town of Newburgh.

As a result of the letter, Seymour asked the Federal Bureau of Investigation to look into Moore's death. "One must start from the assumption that Mr. Hogan's office has thoroughly in-vestigated the homicide aspects of the death of Raymond Moore," Mr. Seymour said. "In view of the serious allegations that have been made, however, we have requested the FBI to initiate an immediate investigation into possible federal civil-rights violations."

The FBI spent two months on this matter, until a generally unnoticed statement by Whitney Seymour appeared in the news-papers: The investigation was concluded, and the FBI had ob-tained a letter of retraction from the guard who had witnessed the beating. Somehow the investigation managed to overlook Kopald, Vanden Heuvel, and myself. Many aspects of the case were never resolved, among them the puzzling question of the undigested food particles.

The case of Raymond Lavon Moore is now legally closed and filed in the official archives, where it is beginning to gather dust.

In a sense, the Board of Corrections' report, entitled "Shuttle to Oblivion," wrote Raymond Lavon Moore's obituary when it said this about his death:

"It must have come as a relief, for who among us could have survived the caged confinement, navigated the labyrinth of justice, endured the endless psychological and physical punishment, and then accepted the medieval dungeon and that final despair of learning that freedom's possibility had expired again with a new warrant by a corrections officer in the court where the whole journey could begin again."

Most of my ventures have brought scant success, and this case seemed no different. Moore was dead; his elderly father grieved; the grand jury had given absolution; the FBI had somehow managed to obliterate a voluntary confession; William vanden Heuvel's well-intentioned promise of prison reform within ninety days had borne no fruit. The suicides continue, and the Tombs is once again more crowded than ever.

But, without being presumptuous, I would like to claim credit for one small success. It came a year later, when a prisoner was found dead in a Brooklyn jail. Dr. Helpern himself crossed the bridge into Brooklyn to personally perform an autopsy— not trusting it to his underlings and not wishing history to repeat itself. A rare and unusual journey for him these days. This time, his findings culminated in an indictment of the prison guards for the slaying of this inmate.

I retain the strange but firm conviction that, had there been a little more humility and less concern for one's ego in certain quarters, the horrible death of Raymond Lavon Moore would have been avenged by a similar conclusion. More people in high places must learn that someone is looking over their shoulders.

5. THE PANTHER TORTURE CASE—THE NEW HAVEN TRIAL

KROGSTAD: "The law does not concern itself with motives."
NORA: "Then the law must be very stupid."
KROGSTAD: "Stupid or not, if I show this paper to the police, you will be judged according to it."

Henrik Ibsen, A DOLL'S HOUSE

In the late afternoon of May 21, 1969, John Mcroczka, a youthful fisherman, and his companion discovered the dead body of a young, goateed black male partially submerged in a swamplike river bed in Middlefield, Connecticut, not far from New Haven. Shortly thereafter, Durham County's medical examiner, Charles Chace, and several police officers arrived at the scene. They examined the site for clues, photographed the body, and arranged for its removal to the Middletown Hospital morgue, where Coroner Harold Campbell requested Dr. Christie McLeod, the local hospital pathologist, to perform an autopsy.

From her autopsy observations, Dr. McLeod concluded that the man had been killed by two bullets, one entering the left side of the head, and the other the front of the chest. She also noted that a wire hanger was loosely twisted around the deceased's neck; that the surface of the body was covered with a number of blistered second-degree burns; that there were bruises in the left groin and over the right eye; and that there was a finger infection that was at least three days old. Dr. Mc-Leod further stated that death had probably taken place some-time between twelve and twenty-four hours before 8:15 P.M., the time at which she began her autopsy on May 21. She finished this procedure at 4:30 A.M. on the twenty-second. Her in-terpretation as to the time of death was based on the fact that rigor mortis by this time involved all four extremities.

The body was identified as that of twenty-four-year-old Alex Rackley. Only eight hours after discovery of the body, the local police, aided by an informer, arrested a few suspects. Ultimately eight members of the Black Panthers were taken into custody. Among those apprehended was Lonnie McLucas, leader of the New Haven Panthers, who was seized in Salt Lake City. Accord-ing to FBI agent Lynn Tweed, who interrogated him there on June 8, 1969, McLucas said he was on his way to California to be appointed "field director" in charge of all Panther activities on the East Coast from Boston down to the Mason-Dixon line. Tweed claimed McLucas admitted firing a shot into the body of Alex Rackley under orders from George Sams, Jr., who had told the local Black Panthers he had been sent to New Haven by National Headquarters and that he had more authority than anyone else on the East Coast in the Party.

Two months later, Sams was apprehended and insisted that Bobby Seale had ordered the execution of Rackley.

At the preliminary presentation of evidence, the police main-tained Rackley was killed because he was suspected of being a police agent. They revealed he was held captive for a few days in a New Haven apartment, tortured with boiling water, and given a "trial" that the Panthers themselves tape-recorded. The tape was later seized by the police. On the night of the murder, Sams allegedly turned the victim loose in the woods with instructions to be careful because of Minute Men in the area. Sams then handed a .45-caliber pistol to Warren Kimbro, another suspect, and said, "Ice him—it's an order from National Headquarters."

Flatly contradicting this view of the affair, the New Haven Panthers claimed that Rackley, originally from Florida, had been a member in good standing and that his death was engineered by Sams, who, they contended, was the one secretly working for the police. They also said Sams had spent almost four years in two New York mental institutions. The Eastern Correctional Institution (now called The Catskill Reformatory), where Sams had been confined from 1961 until November 1964, confirmed that he was "an alleged dangerous mental defective."

It wasn't long before a series of indictments were handed down against the eight Panthers, who were jailed and held without bail for a year before finally being brought to trial.

In the early spring of the next year, while the pretrial hearings in the superior court in New Haven were in progress, I was retained by the lawyers for the defense to analyze and interpret the autopsy findings on Alex Rackley. Up to this point, I had only a fuzzy idea of the entire affair, obtained from a brief reading of the news accounts. I didn't think that I could be much help, even after I'd read the autopsy report. The manner of the death seemed cut and dried, and the remainder of the autopsy findings did not appear to be of any relevance in the preparation of a defense. In addition, by the time I was scheduled to meet with the attorneys, Sams and Kimbro had already confessed, pleaded guilty to second-degree murder, and had agreed to appear as witnesses for the prosecution. What help could I be? But I agreed to try, not really sure of my motives.

So I drove to New Haven, but I had overestimated the driving time. Catherine Roraback, the Connecticut attorney in whose office I was to meet with the lawyers engaged in the defense of the New Haven Black Panthers, was not due in her office until 9:00 A.M. The office was closed and I was left with more than a half hour to wait. The building was located on a street bordering the New Haven green. It was a remarkably clear, balmy spring morning, so I crossed over to the green and relaxed on one of the benches, breathing in the crisp air away from New York. The warming feeling of the sun, and the scene itself, evoked nostalgia for the many springs during my youth when I had been at other village greens, which had always symbolized to me the revolutionary origins of our country (and which no doubt says something about the lure New England has for a Jewish boy from New York). My elementary history lessons were all accompanied by pictures of Revolutionary soldiers on village greens. Suddenly the connection between this historical tradition and the coming trial came into focus: I identified these Panthers with those early Revolutionary soldiers; both had wanted to get "the man" off their backs.

A half hour later, in attorney Roraback's cramped, almost boxlike office, sparsely furnished with a battered wooden desk with papers piled high, a small table, and some wooden chairs, facing the one window looking out on New Haven's tradition-enriched green, I was introduced to the defense attorneys. This group was as varied in appearance, political persuasion, and background as one could ever meet. First there was Catherine Roraback, a handsome, energetic woman who seemed to be of New England pioneer stock. She is nationally known for her legal arguments in the Yale-New Haven Hospital case concerning the right to dispense birth-control information and contraceptive devices, a case she fought all the way to the Supreme Court of the United States and lost. The court upheld Connecticut's nineteenth-century law. In the current trial, she was primarily responsible for the defense of Erica Huggins, deputy chairman of the Black Panther Party; Frances Carter; and Mar-

garet Hudgins. Next was Theodore Koskoff, representing a legal
team that comprised his son and himself. He is portly, gray-
haired, highly experienced, and a locally respected attorney. He
had most recently been in the news because of his defense of
the infamous Danbury bank robbers, those Keystone Kop throw-
backs who set a fire in one part of town and robbed a bank
in another. Theodore Koskoff was the main counsel for Lonnie
McLucas. Edward Flynn, lawyer for George Edwards, was a
tall, thin, sandy-haired man, full of Irish charm and wit, and the
regular legal counsel for several of the local police associations.
There were two recent law graduates, idealistic and studious in
appearance: Scott Melville, defending Rose Smith, and David
Rose, acting as the East Coast representative of Charles Gary
of California, the main lawyer for Bobby Seale (the real target
of the trial). Gary had previously handled the defense of Huey
Newton and the major Panther cases on the West Coast.

This defense-strategy conference met almost at the very moment when the state's attorney, Arnold Markle, was petitioning
Superior Court Judge Harold Mulvey to prevent a joint trial
of all the defendants. His immediate aim was to separate the
prosecution of Lonnie McLucas from the others. Markle had
already worked out deals with Warren Kimbro and George
Sams. For the moment, therefore, McLucas was the state's main
concern and the most vulnerable of the defendants; he seemed
the easiest to convict, and Markle hoped to link Bobby Seale
to the torture and murder of Alex Rackley through McLucas.

Koskoff went off to appear before Judge Mulvey with a wide-
ranging series of arguments challenging Markle's motion. He
argued that separate trials would result in an unconstitutional
denial of a fair trial. He suggested that whichever defendant
was to be tried first (in this case it was to be his client McLucas)
would not have the benefit of the testimony of his alleged cocon-
spirators. The remaining defendants would hesitate to testify in

advance of their own trials and would most likely invoke the Fifth Amendment. Perhaps even more pertinent was the argument that separate trials would mean that all of the essential evidence of the first or earlier trials would be publicized and make fair trials for the remaining defendants an impossibility. It was also argued that a single, joint trial, the state's attorney's arguments notwithstanding, was called for under Connecticut law. Separate trials might be in order only if the defense requested them.

Another defense lawyer claimed that if there were separate trials, the state would have the power to grant partial immunity to some of the defendants. This would force them to testify against one another or else be held in contempt (as had already happened to one of them, Frances Carter). Separate trials would also burden the defendants with increased costs, since each lawyer would have to be present at every trial and would need to buy five times as many transcripts.

Despite these arguments, Judge Mulvey granted the state's attorney's motion for a separate trial for McLucas and announced that this would begin on June 9. The specific charges against McLucas were these: kidnaping, resulting in the death of Alex Rackley; conspiracy to murder; and binding (tying up a victim) with intent to commit a crime.

After the usual introductions, we got down to the serious business at hand. They told me that an arrangement had been made with State's Attorney Markle for me to have a firsthand look at the microscopic slides made from the many skin wounds on Rackley's body. Anticipating this possibility, I had brought my microscope along, knowing that one would not be available at the state's attorney's office in the Superior Court Building. I was also to have an opportunity to study the set of photographs taken in the swampy area and a series of color photographs and X-ray pictures made at the autopsy. The time set for the review of this material was 2:00 P.M.

At lunch, the defense attorneys had several questions to ask. I cautioned them that up to this point I had studied the autopsy findings without the availability of any of the hard facts concerning the background and circumstances surrounding the death. Dr. McLeod's examination was thorough and well performed and seemed to have been completely, accurately, and truthfully recorded. All the relevant tests had been done, and all that remained was for me to look at the slides and photographs. With that caveat in mind, the defense attorneys flung a series of questions at me. From these I selected only those for which the autopsy findings could provide a reasonable answer. The first question related to the accuracy of Dr. McLeod's estimate of the approximate time of Rackley's death. The lawyers wanted to know if death could have occurred considerably earlier or later than the range of her estimate. If one could demonstrate that a significant variation existed from her pretrial testimony, it could be used to challenge the credibility of some of the state's witnesses. From the evidence available, it seemed that rigor mortis was complete when she examined the body at 8:15 P.M. on Monday, May 21; Dr. McLeod had placed the time of death approximately twelve to twenty-four hours prior to the delivery of the body to the hospital. I said that the most anyone could reasonably modify this estimate was to extend the period from twenty-four to thirty-six hours. I would not reduce it below the twelve-hour limit set by Dr. McLeod.

I explained to the lawyers that, even under the best conditions, estimating the time of death is a hazardous undertaking. There could be slight (or sometimes significant) errors, particularly when using rigor mortis as a guide. The speed of onset and the rate of disappearance of rigor mortis can be altered by variations in the temperature of the body at the time of death and the temperature of the surrounding area, and in this case by the length of time and the degree of submersion of the body in the water where it was found, as well as the water's temperature and the speed of its flow. Rackley's physical condition at the time he was killed could also influence the onset of rigor mortis. Considering all these variables and the fact that rigor mortis was present in both the upper and lower extremities, the magnitude of a reasonable variation from the original estimate would not be sufficient to challenge the state's view of the sequence of events. Unlike Perry Mason, whose experts almost always are capable of fixing the time of death within a half hour of its occurrence (as a result of which Mason solves so many cases), I was in no position to do this. I illustrated this with a public humiliation I had suffered as a medical examiner back in Westchester County.

Once in my entire career, I momentarily relaxed my guard and categorically announced an exact time of death. It was in the case of the still unsolved murder of a prominent Yonkers labor leader. At the scene of the crime, I noted that the crystal of the wrist watch worn by the slain man was broken and that the watch had stopped. The amount of rigor mortis already set in coincided with the time on the watch. Feeling reasonably certain about the time of death, I responded to the pressure exerted on me by the New York *Times* Westchester reporter, Merril Folsom, and officially gave him an exact time. He published this as a direct quote from me. To my embarrassment, four reliable witnesses appeared and swore they had seen the deceased alive at least six hours after the time I had given for his death. Merril Folsom couldn't resist reporting this, and made sure my error would not go unnoticed. He looked upon it as a huge joke. At the time, I took a dim view of his sense of humor.

Attorney Flynn brought up for consideration Dr. McLeod's

statement that the blisters on Rackley's body were anywhere from two to seven days old. My opinion in this matter was not in conflict with Dr. McLeod's. It seemed that we were getting nowhere until Theodore Koskoff had a question that related only to the defense of Lonnie McLucas. He asked if I could tell which shot had been fired first and what the reasonable survival times were for each of these injuries if incurred independently. Koskoff didn't say why he wanted this information; I assumed he did not wish to influence my opinion. There were two bullet wounds; either one alone was lethal. Each was capable of causing almost instantaneous death. The bullet wound of the skull, with massive damage to the brain and complete disintegration of the vital centers that control the heartbeat and breathing, was entirely incompatible with life and could cause death in a matter of moments. The chest wound perforated the heart, producing massive internal hemorrhage, which could also lead to a very rapid death.

I explained to Koskoff how difficult it is (on the sole basis of the anatomic evidence) to determine precisely which was the first shot. Nevertheless I believed that, from the evidence immediately available, the head wound was the first. This opinion was based upon the strong probability that bullet-incurred brain damage had caused death before a bullet entered the chest. If Rackley had been alive when the second bullet penetrated the heart and lungs, there still would have been sufficient blood pressure, blood flow, and time to allow the leaking blood to enter the bronchus (this was also part of the bullet-track wound) and well up into the mouth or at least into a portion of the lungs. At autopsy, no red blood was described in these areas.

After listening patiently, Koskoff revealed that the state's evidence, based on statements obtained from Warren Kimbro and George Sams, indicated the head wound was indeed the first and was produced by a shot fired by Kimbro. The chest wound was the second shot, fired by Lonnie McLucas. He then asked: if several minutes had passed, could Rackley have been dead by the time of the second shot? I answered that if these were the facts, then it was a reasonable assumption that Rackley was dead before McLucas shot him. Subsequently, this opinion of mine became the keystone in the strategy for the defense of McLucas.

We finished lunch, and Catherine Roraback directed me to the State's Attorney's office in the courthouse to examine the slides and photographs. My final, written report to the defense counsel was based upon Dr. McLeod's autopsy report, her pretrial testimony, and the material studied in the state's attorney's office.

After returning home that evening, I began preparing a written report. Robby, my younger son, then sixteen years old and deeply committed to the civil-rights struggle, waited impatiently for me to finish what I was doing, so that he could receive a firsthand account.

My written analysis of the case was mainly directed toward the McLucas defense; the minor points of difference from Dr. McLeod's interpretations of the time of death, and the number of days required for the development of the finger infection, were of little consequence and in no way could be used to discredit the state's case against the other defendants. In writing this report I now was fortified with the defense attorney's account of the circumstances leading up to the shooting, and the events surrounding the death itself, along with my examination of the microscopic slides, photographs, and X-ray pictures. The photographs were of little value. Their quality and the lack of sharp close-up detail precluded their use for any scientific examination of the time and cause of the injuries; they had no value as evidence. Their introduction at the trial by the prosecution could only be sensational, an attempt to prejudice the jurors emotionally against the defendants. I understood that the defense was going to object to their introduction as evidence. In this sense, my negative evaluation of these pictures might be helpful in influencing the judge to rule against their introduction. The main thrust of the report emphasized the strong probability that the first shot fired by Kimbro had killed Rackley almost instantaneously and that the victim was in all reasonable likelihood dead by the time McLucas fired the shot into the chest several minutes later.

The report finished, I sat down with Robby and began relating the details of the day's events. Upon reaching that point in the story at which Kimbro and McLucas had fired successive shots, my son almost jumped out of his seat. "I don't believe it! How could you be so sure? It can't have happened that way." Robby looked upon the Panthers as sort of modern-day Robin Hoods. The "movement" had to be clean to gain his full support. The shock of hearing the reality that the Panthers might have actually tortured and killed momentarily shattered his beliefs in any of their existing virtues and made it impossible for him to understand or condone my continued participation in their defense. "No, the whole thing from beginning to end must have been a frame-up." When he finally realized that what I had told him was true, he asked: "Are you still going to be in the case?"

I said, "Yes," without any hesitation. But inwardly, for a second or two, I wasn't so sure. I did have doubts about my position; I was coming to the aid of a man who had admittedly shot another. But I felt there was something different about this case: It wasn't the common-or-garden-variety criminal act. This case was basically political. Everything about it was colored by this—the public's reaction to the charges and the trial, the judge's attitude toward the defendant, and the state's motives for prosecuting. I had begun to see that the state was not really after

McLucas or Sams or Kimbro; they wanted Bobby Seale. Everything that was going to happen in the courtroom was irrevocably tied to politics; the morality and ethics of the Panthers was going to be weighed against the established standards of behavior and law of our society.

What it came down to was: whose law and order were we talking about? At the time of the McLucas trial, even I didn't fully appreciate the extent of the difference between the two value systems. Angela Davis crystallized my feelings about the conflict of the systems when she commented, after her acquittal on the charge of supplying guns for a courtroom shoot-out in California: "The only fair trial would have been no trial at all."

I tried to explain all this to Robby. According to the Panthers' appraisal of their situation, they are at war with an oppressor state. Out of this arise their values, their morality, and their actions. Hence an informer in their ranks is a traitor, to be despised and liquidated. Their evaluation of their microcosmos and their behavior are basically no different from that of the IRA, past and present, who also execute informers, assassinate and tar and feather collaborators; no different from the Jews in the early days of the struggle for a Jewish homeland in Palestine when the Stern Gang, a group of terrorist Jews, also killed informers; no different from Africa when the Mau Mau, led by Kenyatta, killed informers and brutalized their English oppressors; or from the small bands of American rebels during the American Revolutionary period who likewise killed those in their ranks who informed. In every instance, these were regarded by one side in the struggle as essential acts, and those who executed these acts were regarded as heroes (moral considerations notwithstanding). Many Irish and Jews in this country look back upon their revolutionary terrorist counterparts as heroes, and exempt them from their own current sense of morality and standards, but, at the same time, these ethnic groups are blind to the obvious analogy and regard the Panthers as ruthless gangsters. Kenyatta, the head of the Mau Mau, once imprisoned and condemned by the British and world opinion, is now the chief of state in his liberated Kenya. I made these remarks to Robby not to condone the criminal acts, the murders, the killings, but to provide him with some greater measure of understanding. Within this context, for anyone to pass judgment is to condemn himself.

What were McLucas' motives in this crime? Was it for political goals or for personal or vengeful gain? What was his intent? Did he go into this wholeheartedly, or was he intimidated by Sams? Did he really intend to kill? Would he have shot Rackley if Rackley had been alive? Did he know Rackley was dead when he fired the shot? Was Rackley an informer, or a patsy set up by Sams? Was Sams the real villain? Was he really acting sincerely on behalf of the national leadership of the Black Panther Party? Did he have doubts? Or was the entire plot provoked by the police with the connivance of Sams to get at Bobby Seale and destroy the Panthers?

I told Robby that there were too many imponderables, too many shades of gray in this case for me not to lend my support. Let the trial itself attempt to answer some of these questions. I was going to give McLucas the benefit of the doubt, and all the help I could.

The trial began on July 14, but it was not until August 20 that I was called to testify. The intervening weeks had been consumed by many defense-counsel motions, jury selection, the presentation of the prosecution's case, and the first part of the defense's case.

Prior to the jury selection, Theodore Koskoff had moved before Judge Mulvey for dismissal of the trial because the jurors' panel in the State of Connecticut was limited to registered voters. This meant that many citizens of the state, and especially the minority peoples, were excluded from possible jury duty, and for this reason it would be impossible to produce an "impartial jury of his [McLucas'] peers." The motion was overruled. A jury was finally seated and consisted of ten whites and two blacks, and was composed equally of men and women.

The opening of the trial, strangely, coincided with Bastille Day, and was recognized locally in New Haven with a display of some of the trappings of the French Revolution: The French tricolor floated in the breeze above City Hall. Inside the courtroom, a young woman emphasized the revolutionary aspects of the trial with a literary allusion: she sat knitting in the front row of the spectators' section in conscious imitation of Madame Defarge.

Kimbro and Sams were the star witnesses for the prosecution, having turned state's evidence after pleading guilty of second-degree manslaughter. Kimbro had changed his original plea of not guilty to guilty only after a visit from his brother, who was a member of the police force in Florida. On the stand both testified to what was already common knowledge, publicized over the news media. Kimbro failed to corroborate Sams's repeated claim that the initial orders to kill Rackley originated with Bobby Seale, presumably when he had last visited New Haven. Sams also swore he had been ordered to kill Fred Hampton and if necessary even Lonnie McLucas.

On cross-examination by Koskoff, many of Sams's inconsistencies and contradictory statements were uncovered. Among these was testimony in court that two shots had been fired; previously he had said eight or nine shots had been fired. He also admitted to having smoked marijuana and being "high" at the time of the shooting.

The only medical witness called by the prosecution was Durham County's medical examiner, Dr. Charles Chace. On direct examination he stated that Rackley had been shot twice and that either one of the bullet wounds could have been fatal. He did not specify the possible length of survival after each shot. The prosecution never pressed him for this information. The defense counsel carefully avoided cross-examining Dr. Chace on this point. They did not wish to give State's Attorney Markle the slightest hint as to the strategy of the defense or call Markle's attention to the oversight in Chace's testimony.

I did not understand why Dr. McLeod had not been called to testify. She had performed the autopsy and had stated on record, in pretrial testimony, that Rackley could have survived for several hours after the head wound. The seeming failure of the state's attorney to anticipate the content of my testimony, and how this was to be used by the defense, proved damaging to the state's case.

During the presentation of the prosecution's case Judge Mulvey sustained Koskoff's objections to the introduction of the six color slide photos of Rackley's body as evidential exhibits to be shown to the jury, on the grounds that this material would be "inflammatory" and prejudicial to the defendant. In Koskoff's arguments supporting his objection to these photos, he included my opinion that these pictures were of such a poor quality that they could serve no useful purpose in clarifying any of the facts regarding the time of death or cause of the bodily injuries. His was one of the few defense objections or motions not overruled or denied by Judge Mulvey.

As the trial progressed, I was struck by the air of informality and friendliness on the part of the court personnel and the general feeling of relaxation in the courtroom itself. I had never experienced anything like it in my recent years of appearing in the various courts in New York City. In New York the court buildings are forbidding, stern, impersonal, and poorly maintained, making one wonder how any justice could be dispensed with compassion. In New Haven, despite the air-conditioned courtroom and the replacement of the windows with bulletproof glass, one could still sense the bees buzzing around outside. In the hall leading to the courtroom a long line of young civil-rights activists, boys, girls, black and white, in all types of informal dress, waited patiently for their turn to be allowed in to view the proceedings. This day in particular I was told the line was unusually long because it was known that following my testimony, Lonnie McLucas was to take the stand as a witness in his own behalf.

After being sworn in as witness, I noticed Lonnie McLucas sitting somewhat to my left across from me. This was the first time I had seen him in person. In any of the cases in which I have testified on their behalf as a medical expert I have always been careful to avoid a personal meeting with the defendants. Not infrequently, the cross-examining attorney will ask if I am personally acquainted with, or have had any discussions or conversations with, or if I have ever met, the defendant. It is essential, to avoid being accused of bias, to be able to answer no. It also allows for a more dispassionate view of the facts in the case.

McLucas was conservatively dressed in a gray suit, white shirt, and tie. This typified Koskoff's strict formalistic, conservative, and legalistic approach to the defense, very different from a political defense, in which the lifestyle of the defendant is flamboyantly displayed, if not deliberately flaunted, in court.

Koskoff began by asking me the facts of my training, education, and experience as a pathologist. After the first two questions along these lines, State's Attorney Markle indicated that Koskoff could dispense with this line of questioning; he was, he said, willing to accept my qualifications as an expert without taking the time to go into all the details. On the surface, Markle's act seemed a magnanimous gesture. Actually he probably wanted to prevent the jury from having access to the credentials, which might unduly impress them in the event he wished to challenge my testimony. Koskoff was not taken in by this. He thanked Markle but continued questioning me on every detail of my career relevant to my expertise in this case. This was also the only opportunity Koskoff would have to record my qualifications, and this was essential if in the future an appeal to a higher court would be required.

This line of questions completed, Koskoff then asked if I had had an opportunity to study the autopsy record, the slides, and the photographs of the deceased Rackley. I answered, "Yes." Koskoff then asked, "Would you please disclose the nature of the two bullet wounds and give an opinion if you can as to how soon death would have occurred after the first shot; the shot fired by Kimbro—that is, the head wound." I described the two wounds and then answered that I thought death would have occurred "almost instantly" after the first shot. Why did I think so? Koskoff asked.

With this question, and with the permission of the judge, I stepped down from the witness box and stood in front of a large sketch of the brain mounted on an easel. This simplified sketch depicted the course of the bullet, where it had struck the brain, and the area of brain damage. The sketch and permission to show it had been previously arranged for by Koskoff. I carefully explained the sketch to the court, with particular emphasis on the fact that the vital centers that controlled the heartbeat and breathing had been in the area completely destroyed by the bullet wound. With the destruction of these main control centers, no stimuli could reach the heart and the lungs, and these organs would cease functioning. Death would then be instantaneous. I went back to the witness box.

Koskoff then asked his key question. "In other words, Dr. Spain, with these facts at your disposal, and on the assumption that several minutes had elapsed between the first shot and this

second shot, would you conclude that it was reasonable to assume that Rackley was dead before McLucas shot him?"

"Yes."

This concluded the direct examination.

Markle, from whom I expected a vigorous and prolonged attempt to challenge this assumption, surprised me by ignoring
this entirely. After the usual routine questions from him as to
whether I had known the defendant, how many discussions I
had had with the attorney, and so forth, he asked if in my opinion it was possible for a non-physician, a layman such as Lonnie
McLucas, to recognize when a man had just died. I responded,
"Yes," but qualified it with the remark that the ability to do
so would vary with a number of circumstances. Markle then
asked, "You are talking about medical death, Doctor, are you
not? Not legal death." As I was responding to this with "I don't
understand the question," Koskoff was already on his feet ob-
jecting to the question. The judge said it would not be necessary for him to rule on this, because, as far as he was concerned,
I had already given a satisfactory answer, and permitted no further questioning along these lines.

Markle had no other questions. I was dismissed. Cross-
examination had lasted only about five minutes. A recess was
declared for motions to be heard by opposing attorneys. While
I was waiting outside the courtroom for Koskoff to appear,
Markle came along. As he approached me, I told him that I
was surprised by the brevity of his cross-examination. He said,
"I had previously checked you out with the District Attorney
of Westchester County, and I know when it's best not to stick
my neck out." I thanked him for his compliment. I think,
though, that he had behaved in the smartest manner possible.
Some lawyers, on the verge of victory, fail because they overtry
their cases. One question too many can be their undoing. Markle
knew it would be best not to tangle with me on an issue where

he was no expert, especially when he had no medical consultant immediately available; and it was no longer legally possible, at this stage, for him to introduce one into the trial. Although he had not anticipated this line of testimony, he now attempted to recoup this lost ground with the best possible tactic under the circumstances. He ignored the portion of my testimony concerning the probability of Rackley's death before the second shot, to diminish its importance in the minds of the jury.

Now that he understood a major thrust of Koskoff's ultimate defense strategy, Markle aimed at neutralizing it. He challenged me on the ability of a layman like McLucas to recognize that Rackley was dead.

The diagnosis and criteria of death have become a major matter of public concern because of medical advances in the transplant of organs and the development of artificial life-support systems. Great public apprehension has developed over the diagnosis of death, and heretofore unresolved and neglected moral, legal, and ethical questions have become the subject of theological, medical, and judiciary debate.

In the past it was simple. Death was when the doctor diagnosed it as such, and there seems to have been no legal distinction about how death should be defined. The courts in the past have been concerned mainly with the proof of death (evidence taken as "judicial notice") and proof of the time of death. The fact of death may also be established by witnesses or physicians, preferably the latter. In brief, it appears that the courts accept common-knowledge facts as evidence of death. Until organ transplant became a reality, the public rarely questioned the previous practices in the definition of death. New techniques have necessitated more precise determinations of the moment of death, using such instruments as an electroencephalograph to determine the presence or absence of electrical activity in the brain. The absence of such activity is now used to indicate death.

When Markle asked whether I was referring to medical death or legal death, he was obviously playing upon the recent controversy and public attitudes in this matter. However, these were technicalities that had no relevance to the recognition of death in this case; it is accepted fact that most people can readily recognize death.

When McLucas took the stand, he was questioned at length by Koskoff in order to develop the idea that the defendant was unaware of Sams's murderous intentions toward Rackley, and participated in the killing only out of tremendous fear of Sams. In connection with this, Koskoff asked McLucas: "How did he [Rackley] appear to you as he fell [after Kimbro's shot]?" "Dead," McLucas replied, and then said Sams sent him back into the swamp "to make sure he was dead." And he interpreted this to mean he was supposed to fire another shot: "I went to where the body lay and aimed the flashlight and fired."

Koskoff asked, "Did you look at the body?"

McLucas: "I saw his eyes were open and they were glazed."

"How did he appear to you?"

McLucas: "Dead. Dead."

On cross-examination of McLucas, the state's attorney vigorously attempted to destroy any impression the defendant might have made on the jury that he was an unwilling participant, that he did not know Rackley was to be killed, that he had fired the shot only out of fear of Sams and then only because he thought the victim was already dead. At one point, Markle scornfully demanded to know from McLucas how Sams could have forced him to do anything when he (McLucas) was holding "the business end of a .45." Markle: "You didn't turn the gun on Sams and say, 'I am not shooting anyone,' did—." McLucas broke in, and said that there was a rifle in the car. Markle, however, brought out that Sams and Kimbro were not in the car but outside, unarmed.

The case went to the jury. The verdict came on the sixth day, the longest any Connecticut jury had ever deliberated. Lonnie McLucas was found guilty of only one charge, the conspiracy one, for his role in the Alex Rackley slaying, but was acquitted on the other three charges, all of which carried heavier penalties, ranging from twenty-five years to death. The maximum sentence the twenty-four-year-old Black Panther chieftain now faced was fifteen years. Upon hearing the verdict, McLucas openly expressed joy. But, outside, a small group of Panther supporters and activists were chanting, "Free Lonnie!" "Protest the racist frame-up!" However, most demonstrators were relieved that he had been found guilty on the least serious of all the charges. Koskoff expressed satisfaction with the result and believed McLucas had been given a fair trial.

After the jury was officially discharged, one of the jurors, who preferred to remain anonymous, told the press: "Lonnie McLucas is a gentle man. He is no detriment to society. It is his testimony that freed him, not his defense. He was as honest as the FBI and the New Haven police." Credibility is the key word. After all is said and done, most cases revolve on whom the jury decides to believe.

Why did this juror and the others attach more credibility to McLucas' words than to Sams's? Probably because Sams had a stake in aiding the state's case. Many suspected a deal had been made between Sams and Markle. Although there was no factual evidence to support this, a later event tended to reinforce these suspicions. Sams had served only two years of his sentence when an unusual request was made by State's Attorney Markle to the Connecticut Board of Pardons. He asked for Sams's release on the grounds that the prisoner had been of service to the state in testifying against Seale and was entitled to every consideration. In the period between the McLucas case and Markle's application to the Connecticut Board, Sams had been trotted out of prison once again as the star witness for the state. This time it was part of an effort to show that Seale was the over-all "boss" who ordered the "contract" for the slaying of Rackley. Seale was tried and found not guilty. Of unusual interest was a statement by the former police chief of New Haven, James F. Ahern, in which he insisted there was never any "solid evidence" to link Bobby Seale to the murder of Rackley and that he was "astonished" when the Panther chairman was indicted. The McLucas case was a test between the credibility of Sams and that of McLucas; and the recent disillusionment of the public with hired informers was probably what turned the tide in favor of McLucas.

Still unanswered by the trial and the weeks of testimony and the verdict of the jury were a number of the basic questions I had raised in my discussions with Robby before the trial. Was McLucas really a "shnook," or was he a willing, active partner in the entire sordid affair? Was Rackley an innocent patsy set up by Sams, or was he in reality a paid agent of the police sent in to spy and inform on the Panthers? Was Sams a vicious mental defective, a psychopath who, as an adventurer, happened to become involved with the Panthers, or was he for one reason or another prompted to act as an *agent provocateur* for the state? These questions remain incompletely answered after the trial, and perhaps never will be resolved.

In the light of my personal experience and exposure to recent so-called political cases, I have gained a distinct impression that a curious paradox exists. Where certain clear acts have been committed within a situation having political overtones, the defendants have in the past few years a better chance of acquittal, or sentencing with a lesser degree of punishment, than if the same crime had been committed devoid of a political setting.

Judges and juries have become highly cautious because of close public scrutiny of these cases by the many civil-rights, civil-libertarian, and minority political organizations. Or perhaps it is because crimes committed within a political context arise out of a social motivation rather than vengeance, hate, or desire for personal material gain.

How to render justice where crimes stemming from the highest motives conflict with established, historically tested law is, at least to me, an insoluble problem. I find myself switching sides, depending on the subtleties of each case. Truly objective and irrevocable moral standards as guidelines do not exist.

6. A BAG OF BONES—MURDER IN BALTIMORE

"Elementary, my dear Watson."

A. Conan Doyle

When Harold Buchman, a Baltimore attorney, called to ask me to examine a "bag of bones" for him in May 1971, I took the request in stride. I've had to do a lot of bizarre—as well as gory—things as medical examiner, and it was the political rather than the physical aspect that piqued my interest in Buchman's case. He was defending Arthur Turco, a white "radical" lawyer from the North accused of masterminding the murder of a black youth. The State of Maryland believed that Turco was a Black Panther (an unlikely possibility, since no whites have ever been allowed in the Party) who had discovered a police informer in the Panther ranks and had him tortured and killed. It was the Alex Rackley story all over again, except for two interesting twists: the alleged murderer was white, and the corpse consisted of little more than bare bones.

Buchman told me that the events leading up to Turco's arrest began sometime in July of 1969, when a twenty-year-old black youth named Eugene Leroy Anderson vanished. Anderson had supposedly been hired by the Baltimore Panthers to paint their quarters, and it was soon after this contact that his disappearance was reported. A search was conducted for several months but proved fruitless. The police seemed convinced that the disappearance was murder and that the murder was a Panther action—thanks to an informer. The informer linked Turco to the plot, despite the fact that he was not a Baltimore resident but was a New York lawyer. At the time Anderson was reported missing, Turco was in Baltimore defending several Panthers on a robbery charge. Assistant State's Attorney Caplan—working on the informer's reports—insisted that Turco had been present at Panther headquarters while Anderson was beaten, tortured with a hot knife, forcibly held in custody for several days, and finally killed with a shotgun in a southwest-Baltimore park—and that it was all at Turco's instigation.

But Caplan couldn't make these charges until a year later; in the absence of a body, Anderson's fate couldn't be determined and no charges could be brought against the suspects. In 1970, bones were found lying on a long board in a Baltimore park, by someone taking a leisurely stroll. Caplan was ready to move; he indicted seventeen Panthers, ex-Panthers, and Panther supporters, plus Turco, for the "torture murder" of Anderson. Three of the alleged participants were offered immunity from prosecution and turned state's evidence, incriminating Turco.

I was intrigued by Buchman's story. How could the state possibly charge Turco with all these atrocities if all they had in the way of physical evidence was (as Buchman kept calling it) "a bag of bones"? Buchman gave me to understand that there were precious few bones in that bag and that the remains had initially been identified as someone else. Could I come down and examine the bones? I could.

When I was called into the case, Turco had been held in the Baltimore City Jail without bail since April 1970 and would continue to be so through the time his case went to trial, on

June 14, 1971. He and one other of all those indicted remained
charged with a capital crime. Charles Wyche, the man accused
of the actual shooting of Anderson, had been recently acquitted
and the court had dropped or reduced charges against all the
others but Turco and Panther Eddie Conway. Conway, at the
time of Turco's trial, was already serving a life-plus-thirty-year
sentence on these charges; he had asked the court that Turco
be allowed to defend him at his impending trial. The request
was disallowed, and Conway refused to show up at his own
trial. Conway was put into an isolation cell, and the warden
seized all of Turco's books and papers to prevent him from
working on Conway's defense. Conway was tried and found
guilty *in absentia.*

It took a month to obtain permission from the state for me
to examine the "bag of bones." Buchman specifically wanted
to learn if the remnants of the deceased were sufficient to establish without any doubt that these were the bones of Anderson, and he was also anxious to see if the state had sufficient
evidence to determine an unequivocal cause of death. An appointment had been made for me to review all the material at
the medical examiner's office in Baltimore. The Baltimore medical examiner had one of the best reputations in the country.
Dr. Russell Fisher, head of the department, and his associates,
especially Dr. Werner Spitz, were well known to me through
their fine scientific contributions in the field of forensic science.
They were also known to be excellent teachers, and I looked
forward to meeting them.

Once in Baltimore, I went immediately to the scheduled appointment. To reach my destination necessitated walking
through the University of Maryland complex of medical and
dental school buildings. Much change had taken place here over
the previous thirty years, but I was still familiar with the area.
I had gone to medical school here and had lived in this city

for four years. I had returned to this spot just once in the long
interval since then, and one change in particular stood out:
The University Hospital, with two of its wings completed in my
day, had had separate entrances for the two main races it served
—for the whites a central main entry, and a smaller one off to
the side for the blacks. Now everyone, regardless of race, entered through one main point. As I continued walking in this
site, the number of black student nurses, laboratory technicians,
and other black professional personnel was also in startling contrast to my student days. Then the only blacks employed
scrubbed floors, hauled trash, or carried baggage. These changes,
not enough to prevent militant Panther action, nevertheless
moved me—after this extended absence—probably because I recalled my student training in obstetrics, which consisted of being
sent into the many side and back alleys of Baltimore to deliver
pregnant black women in labor. We had called the method used
"the newspaper technique." The blacks in possession of no linen
for bedding would be instructed in advance at the hospital clinic
to collect and save newspapers for the day of delivery so we
would have something relatively clean for them to lie on. During
these delivery sessions, usually in a one-room shack devoid of
inside toilet facilities or running water, the historic entry of another black child in the world would be witnessed by the entire
family, sometimes consisting of three generations and of ten or
so children and adults. My obstetrical manipulations often were
performed to a background of Negro spirituals hummed by these
spectators. Just as I approached the Medical Examiner Building, I recalled once entering a small, broken-down store in one
of these alleys to get a Coca-Cola. The storekeeper refused to
serve me for fear I was out to trap him into a violation of the
Jim Crow code.

In the lobby of the Medical Examiner Building and engraved
in a marble façade overlooking the entrance was the credo of

this department: WHERE THE ART OF MEDICINE IS PRACTICED
THERE IS ALSO A LOVE OF HUMANITY. This heartened me and
I was certain that the men in this department would extend
their fullest co-operation to me in consummating my assignment.
Dr. Spitz was already waiting for me. After the usual formalities
and some small talk about friends and experiences in common,
he briefed me on the background and the investigatory procedures in this case. He outlined the reasons for the conclusions
reached. I was told that physical anthropologists from the Smithsonian Institution, in nearby Washington—called in by the district attorney—had also studied the skeletal remains and that
their determinations were in accord with the medical examiner's.
The specimens, essential records, X-ray pictures, and pertinent
reports had all been assembled in advance for my personal review. Dr. Spitz then left me alone in a conference room assigned
to my use, where I could study all this material and evidence
undisturbed and at my own pace.

All along, I had felt uneasy that Buchman had, either intentionally or, more likely, because he himself was poorly informed,
misrepresented or underestimated the number of bones recovered by the police. As I saw it now, the skeleton, except for
a few unimportant small bones in the wrists and fingers, was
intact. Buchman had told me that only two or perhaps three
bones had been located—among them a thighbone and the pelvis.
That is why I had thought the evidence would prove far too
scanty to arrive at any definitive conclusions as to exact identity
or cause of death. With the limited evidence I had expected
to see, it would have been possible to determine sex, approximate age and height, and possibly race—but certainly not any
exact identity. With an almost full skeleton, skull and teeth intact, it was now an entirely different ball game.

Buchman was not the first attorney who had supplied me with
incomplete or patently incorrect facts. Many attorneys have

done this consciously and purposefully, and have underrepresented the evidence against their side of the case in order to ensure my acceptance of the assignment. Other times it was because a lawyer was poorly prepared or faced insurmountable obstacles in getting at the necessary information. In this instance Buchman assured me, and I believed him, that he was unaware of the extent of the state's evidence in the matters relating to my consultation.

Dr. Spitz told me that in the early stages of his investigation he was entirely in the dark as to whom these bones represented. Good medical examiners in cases of this sort follow a careful routine that often yields a large number of solutions to these puzzles. The method used is almost comparable to a well-known game I have often played with my children. We used to call it "twenty questions." One participant would pick the name of a famous person and keep it to himself. The other participants would then be limited to asking twenty questions of the one who had picked the name, in order to uncover the name of the unknown celebrity. Experienced players had a set routine to narrow the possible choices with the least number of questions: the first question would identify sex; the next, age; the third, race or ethnic origins. Those who gambled by wasting their first queries on more specific points soon reached their limit and were out of the game. Those who stuck to the routine and only later asked more specific questions often came up with the exact answer. In the beginning, Spitz did the same thing; he used the bones to find out what he could most surely and readily identify: sex, age, and race. Positive identification of a body is usually easy and is most often completed by the police before the corpse arrives at the morgue for autopsy. Where the deceased is at first unknown, clothing, personal papers, appearance, stature, fingerprints, dental work, scars, physical deformities, and so forth are helpful. There were no clothes, no papers, no flesh, no fingerprints; the problem was of a different magnitude. And with only bones remaining, determining cause of death would be at best difficult, if not impossible.

The bones found lying on a long board in the Baltimore park were, except for ligaments, joint cartilage, and a few small fragments of flesh, clean and stripped bare. The animals, insects, rain, and weather had done an almost thorough job. It looked as if the skeleton were being prepared for an anatomy class. The most cursory examination and the most elementary knowledge were sufficient to see that the remains were human. The appearance suggested exposure rather than burial, for a period ranging from three months to one year, probably for a period of warm weather—or so said the Smithsonian anthropologists and the pathologists from the medical examiner's office. I disagreed in only one respect: I would have extended the possible range of how long the individual might have been dead to somewhat more than one year.

As to whether the bones were from a man or a woman, the bones of the pelvis are the most informative. Even the lower part of the back, or sacrum, or the thighbone, or femur, can provide ample proof of sex. In the male, the pelvis is narrower, the bones are thicker and heavier, the attachments for muscles are more prominent, and the holes through which major nerve trunks exit are larger. Also, the relative length of the breast bone is different in the man. All the accepted criteria unequivocally proved this was a male.

Next came the consideration of age. The accuracy of this determination changes with age. In the fetus, it may be fixed with mathematical precision by the appearance of the ossification centers. These are the points of early bone formation. In youth, evidence of age is obtained from the eruption of the teeth as well as by changes in the bone centers. After twenty-five, the ability to accurately estimate age deteriorates sadly. With the material before me and the X-ray pictures of the bones taken by the medical examiners, the findings suggested the unknown must have been between twenty and twenty-four years old.

The search had now narrowed down to a man of about twenty or more. What did he look like? From the skeleton, only general body build and stature can be approximated. These can be calculated by long-tested and reliable formulas derived from relative lengths of the long bones of the extremities. He appeared to have been somewhere between sixty-three and sixty-seven inches tall (5' 3" to 5' 7") and was slight of build and wiry.

Finally I arrived at the touchy question, race. Always at this point the most well-meaning scientist becomes embroiled in a political, cultural, and emotionally muddied controversy. Are there valid racial or ethnic differences? Some deny the existence of race. Some deny any group differences. The fact that differences are recognized among various population groups and that as scientists we talk about them and use these findings for positive research purposes does not make us racists or reactionaries. Even the most ardent women's liberationist will concede the existence of a few obvious physical and biological differences between male and female and admit that these will not alter in the immediate future. The important thing, though, is that these distinctions should offer no reason for considering one group as inferior to the other and should certainly not justify oppression or the assignment of less quality to the course of their lives.

At any rate, the anthropologists from the Smithsonian stuck their collective necks out and risked the wrath of some of the emotionally charged progressive forces in the community by suggesting that the "relatively long shins and forearms, small pelvis, straight long-bone shafts, form and projection of teeth" indicated Negro race, and that other details, "as a rather small, prominent nose, suggest rather definite white mixture also, as in many American Negroes."

The choice had been reduced considerably—or at least it seemed so on the surface. One only had to connect these determinatives with one mysteriously missing black male of about twenty who was slight of build, wiry, and somewhere about five feet five inches tall. Simple; but where to begin, and where to go from there. The mobility of black youth is well known, and Baltimore enjoys a population of men fitting this description in the hundreds, if not in the thousands.

From certain bone changes, it was also concluded that the deceased had been anemic in childhood and may have suffered from a minor variant of sickle-cell anemia. At one time he must have incurred a severe injury to the bones in the region of the right side of his nose. These observations were of no further help in the identification process.

I now studied the critical clues, the ones that in the absence of all other data might once and for all decisively end the quest.

This was the condition of the teeth and the nature of any dental work. Dental identification now rivals fingerprints as a proved, practical system of identification. Often these two systems supplement each other. It is axiomatic to a pathologist that no unidentified body should ever be removed from the morgue without a complete record of the teeth and without X-ray pictures of the upper and lower jaws from several angles. A description of residual dentition, fillings, dentures, and other relevant changes should be preserved. All modern medical examiners employ, as integral members of their staffs, dentists who are experts in dental forensic matters, and they are always called in in cases like this one. If no other information were available as to age, sex, race, appearance, and so on, the evidence in this one area alone could, and often does, solve identity problems.

The modern sleuth is more often finding it rewarding to consult with a dentist who is also versed in forensic affairs. Untold
numbers of murders remain unsolved only because the bodies
remain unidentified: they are either decomposed, mutilated, or
burned beyond recognition. For some time now, detailed analysis of the teeth, the jaws, and the tissues of the mouth have
been utilized to solve problems of identity.

Where no identity problem exists, a visual description of the
oral cavity and its contents will usually suffice for the autopsy
report. In cases with mouth injury, a more exacting examination
is needed for medical-legal purposes. Compensation and insurance claims stemming from trauma to the mouth, jaws, and teeth
can originate from assault, accident, or alleged dental malpractice. Adjudication of these claims must consider not only the
harm to health because of impaired mastication but the emotional effects caused by alteration in one's appearance. This becomes a critical question if the injured one's looks are related
to his means of livelihood.

In mass disasters such as airliner crashes or explosions in
crowded public places, where many bodies are rendered unrec-
ognizable, the rapidity and accuracy with which one can recover
the correct body for burial becomes an urgent matter of compassionate concern for the victims' next of kin. Often, with the
aid of a dental expert, cross elimination between victims is made
possible and can be speeded up. Dental expertise should be invariably utilized even if it means delay in the release of single
bodies, to assure identification of all the bodies. The delay must
be handled with tact and kindness or else it can be disrupted
by conflicts with the authorities, the press, and victims' families.

A most celebrated murder taken from the criminology archives in the city of Boston centered around dental identification. In 1849 the sudden and unexplained disappearance from
Harvard of the famous Professor Parkman aroused a series of

suspicions. A few days later, a block of porcelain teeth and some bone fragments were recovered from the laboratory furnace of Dr. Webster, the professor of chemistry at Harvard and a close associate of Dr. Parkman. Dr. Webster denied any connection with Parkman's disappearance. But the teeth were soon identified by Parkman's dentist as part of a denture he had made for the missing professor, and they still fitted a plaster model of Parkman's jaw on file in the dentist's office. This evidence was presented in court and led to a legal precedent. For the first time in legal history, dental evidence was accepted as proof of an identifiable corpse. Dr. Webster was found guilty, sentenced to death, and hanged.

This year, a former pathology trainee of mine and now a part-time medical examiner acquainted me with a unique identification case of his own. A headless, armless, and legless torso of a white woman was discovered by two sanitation workers as they unloaded a trash can into their truck. The can had been picked up off the street in front of an abandoned and partially burnt-out tenement. The condition of the remains indicated the victim had been dead for no longer than six or seven days. The missing persons bureau was contacted, and the torso was taken to the medical examiner's morgue. The appearance of the breasts, skin, and genitalia suggested the woman was young and had not yet borne any children. The missing persons bureau called several families who had reported a missing female within the past week to obtain information that might be helpful in the identity of this mutilated body. No helpful characteristic scars, deformities, or stigmata of disease were seen on the surface of the torso or on the X-ray pictures of the spinal and pelvic bones. As the internal organs were about to be dissected, a call came from the missing persons bureau relaying the information obtained from one of the families that had responded to their calls. This family had reported a daughter, aged twenty-three, missing for several days, and on questioning for identifying features they told of an examination performed on her uterus by a gynecologist within the past year. The procedure, a hysterogram, consists of injecting fluid material into the cavity of the uterus so that it casts a shadow on an X-ray picture, outlining any abnormalities. In this case it outlined a small tumor with a very unusual configuration projecting into the external cavity. Upon learning this, my friend repeated the same procedure on the uterus removed from the torso. An identical picture was obtained. Such identifications not only help to solve criminal acts but to an extent relieve the already anguished families of prolonged periods of uncertainty and the strain of living with false hope.

There remains, however, one big "if" in dental identification —if it is possible to find where the unknown's dental work was performed. Only then can records be secured for comparison with the findings, and X-ray pictures obtained of the corpse. Recently, however, there has been a growth of comprehensive files of dental records and X-ray pictures.

In his earlier conference with me, Dr. Spitz related how they happened to come upon the vital dental records and X-ray pictures in this case. There were obviously no fingerprints available. After everything else had been done, Dr. Spitz had called in his dental expert.

His consultant in forensic dentistry found a defect on the outer surface of the left side of the lower jaw. This defect was traced, with the aid of X-ray pictures, to connect with an abscess surrounding a tooth and originating from a cavity in that tooth. According to Spitz, a strange and fortuitous coincidence occurred. While conducting his examination, the dentist was reminded of an almost identical abscess and associated jaw damage he had once treated at the University of Maryland Dental Clinic, where he worked and was a member of the faculty.

Immediately he went to the clinic record room and uncovered the case in mind. Comparison of these dental records and the X-ray pictures with those of the unknown produced a perfect match. In both situations there were seventeen cavities in identical locations in the same teeth; both had one cavity that had been capped, and in both the remainder of the cavities were filled with highly characteristic fillings, some of gold. The diseased areas in the lower jaw bone were identical. The name on the clinic chart was Eugene Leroy Anderson, the missing black youth. I re-examined this crucial data and could only come to the same conclusions as had Spitz and the Smithsonian anthropologists.

To this day I am uncertain whether the sequence of events in this identity search was exactly as Dr. Spitz narrated it. Perhaps it was his sense of the dramatic that prompted him to put the steps taken in this investigation in this order. Dr. Spitz, being the intelligent, well-informed, and skilled medical examiner that he is, would have called in his dental expert at the very inception of the search and would not have waited until the completion of all the other determinations. He would have immediately researched the University Dental Clinic records, regardless of any recollection of a similar case by his dental consultant. This dental clinic was the largest and the busiest in the city, and the odds were strong that a young black man would sooner or later have gone to this clinic for dental care. Any astute investigator would have looked at the clinic records, especially when the main aim was to link these bones with Anderson. The authorities knew that Anderson had once been a student at this university. Nevertheless, Spitz's story as he presented it was intriguing, and he deserves credit for a thorough job well done.

Be that as it may, there was no longer any identity question.

The state now possessed a qualified corpse with which Buch-man had to contend at the trial in his defense of Turco.

As for the second and possibly more vital question in the defense of Turco, the cause of death: This, too, became a problem in the absence of any vital organs for study, and in the absence of any significant amount of flesh on the bones. Again, the changes in the bones proved sufficient to arrive at a highly probable conclusion. The left rib had a freshly broken area "as if from a hard blow." But there was no sure way of knowing if this had occurred just before or after death. More important was the discovery of a small elliptical puncture in a similar area of the left sixth rib, two inches from where it joined the breast-bone. This puncture passed through the rib and traveled in a direction that, if it had continued, would have penetrated the heart. I had been informed in the briefing session that shotgun pellets had been found on the board upon which the skeleton had been found resting. The lead in the shotgun pellets was similar in all characteristics to the lead found in the rib at the puncture margins. A .38-caliber bullet was also found on the board in the neck region at the time of discovery. The lead in it differed from that in the ribs. It was regarded by Spitz as unrelated to the cause of death. He concluded that death was probably caused by a shotgun wound of the heart. The second question was resolved, and Buchman now faced a tough trial.

The trial of Turco for the torture murder of Anderson lasted three weeks, and the jury of six men and six women (eight blacks and four whites) could not agree on a verdict. The judge was forced to dismiss the jury and declare a mistrial. The state was not content to let the matter drop even after the Panther who was accused of actually firing the fatal shot was acquitted. A second trial was ordered. Turco was harassed continually while he was in jail awaiting trial. He had been helping prisoners with many of their legal problems and informing them of their civil rights. During a jail rebellion the inmates chose Turco to negotiate with the prison officials and to present their demands. The officials agreed and promised no reprisals or punishment against the participants. Afterward, however, despite these assurances, the warden accused Turco of masterminding the rebellion. He was thrown into a twenty-four-hour lockup with guards posted in front of his cell to prevent anyone from talking to him. Inmates who merely said hello to him were put in isolation. All his personal and legal property was removed and he was denied food until a shocklike state began to develop (Turco is a diabetic). Finally, he was denied visitors and commissary privileges for sixty days.

I was puzzled by the relentless legal pursuit of this white lawyer. My entire past experience had demonstrated very little concern for justice when blacks had been killed, but this did not tally with the vigor with which the state was going after Turco. Mikulicz, the ex-cop who had killed two blacks in cold blood on the streets of Yonkers because he "hate[d] niggers," had never spent a day in jail. The Westchester police and the district attorney's men would refer to killing of a black as "malicious mischief" and look upon it as a minor crime. The killer would be allowed to plead guilty to a lesser charge and get off with a relatively short sentence. I wanted to think that maybe I was out of tune, maybe attitudes had changed drastically, in keeping with some of the improvements that I saw while walking through the grounds of the medical school. But only a year after this I overheard a comment by a captain in the crime-analysis section of the New York City Police Department and I realized nothing had changed. He was explaining the record high of homicides for the week. He said: "You take a poor guy, a black or a Puerto Rican, it's sweltering, he doesn't have an air conditioner, he's sitting on the stoop, he has a few beers, there's no place

to go; then all of a sudden it breaks out in the open; he grabs
a knife and boom—twenty-six stabbings in one week." If the
guy who did it was a poor, sweating s.o.b., then murder was
only malicious mischief.

Why was Turco being leaned on? Because as William
Kunstler (one of Turco's two defense attorneys) put it in his
opening arguments, the real issue is "whether the government
can use its resources to crush a movement of black men and
women."

Kunstler also said the state's evidence would consist of the
most dangerous kind of testimony—the testimony of accomplices
with everything to gain. And indeed this was the only evidence
allowed to come out at the trial: the testimony of those who
had turned state's evidence. There was precious little tangible
evidence.

Perhaps the State of Maryland realized the sketchy weakness
in its case, and that people on juries have become fed up with
the testimony of paid informers or of those who have made
deals with the state. In any case, the State of Maryland finally
allowed Turco to plead to the charge of "accessory after the
fact," and he was given a suspended sentence. His guilty plea
closed the search for the facts of the murder, and no further
material came out at the trial to explain why the state was so
sure it had the right man.

The single-minded pursuit of a Panther sympathizer made me
revise my judgment about how Baltimore had changed. Its buildings might no longer have separate entrances for blacks and
whites, but it still had two kinds of justice.

II

CRIME IS NEVER CLEAR-CUT

1. ALICE CRIMMINS IN WONDERLAND

"Let the jury consider their verdict," the King said for about the twentieth time that day. "No, no," said the Queen. "Sentence first —verdict afterwards." "Stuff and nonsense!" said Alice loudly. "The idea of having the sentence first."

Lewis Carroll, ALICE'S ADVENTURES IN WONDERLAND

On July 14, 1965, Mrs. Alice Crimmins reported her two children missing. She told the police she had last seen her four-year-old daughter, Alice Marie, and her five-year-old son, Edmund, Jr., in their beds at midnight the night before. Edmund Crimmins, Alice's estranged husband, later recalled that on the day his children disappeared the window in their room was open and its screen was on the ground below it, as if someone had broken in. The lamp usually kept on the bureau in front of the window was gone. Mrs. Crimmins had knocked on a neighbor's door to ask if she had seen the children or if they were in her apartment.

A few hours later, Alice Marie's body was found less than a mile from Mrs. Crimmins' Kew Gardens apartment, in Queens. Five days later, Edmund, Jr.'s body was discovered, also within a mile of his home, but in a different spot.

The Queens County medical examiner, Dr. Richard Grimes, had been called to the scene when Alice Marie's body was found. He described in his report the presence of a child's pajama jacket, loosely wrapped around Alice Marie's face. The autopsy was performed by Dr. Milton Helpern, and his report concluded that death was due to asphyxiation by strangulation. Because Edmund, Jr.'s body was partially decomposed from exposure to the hot, humid summer weather, the autopsy findings were inconclusive and the cause of death was never determined.

The detectives assigned to the case conducted a fruitless investigation. There was insufficient evidence against any suspect for a presentment to the grand jury. The public thought they had reached a dead end. The case disappeared from the headlines.

Then, in November 1966—over a year later—an anonymous letter was received by the police. The writer claimed to have seen Mrs. Crimmins "carrying a blanket-wrapped bundle and leading a small boy, walking with a man from the direction of the Crimmins' apartment to a parked car" the night before Alice Marie's body was found. Another investigation was begun. Early in 1968, nearly three years after the discovery of the dead bodies, Alice Crimmins was indicted for the murder of her daughter.

A few weeks after the indictment, I received a call from Martin Baron, who, along with his partner, Harold Harrison, was defending Alice Crimmins. A well-known pathologist in Queens had recommended me. He asked if I would be willing to confer with them on the technical aspects of the autopsy report on Alice Marie. I expressed doubts as to whether I could be of any help, but he insisted on seeing me. I reluctantly agreed and set up an appointment at my office in the hospital.

When they arrived, I asked them for the autopsy report, which they had brought along. I sized up the findings and the lawyers at the same time. They were not just going through the motions;

both were determined to do everything possible for their client. I asked them what help I could possibly be.

Baron, the spokesman for the two, wanted to know if the autopsy findings really proved beyond a reasonable doubt that Alice Marie's death was due to asphyxiation by strangulation. This was an important point, since the indictment against Alice Crimmins listed strangulation as the cause. He also wanted to know if the death could have been a natural one, whether there was any evidence of sexual attack on the body, and what the evidence was for determining the time of death.

Since I couldn't answer these questions without a careful study of the autopsy report, I set up another meeting, cautioning the men that I wasn't committing myself to testifying in court. Baron declared himself agreeable.

Before they left, laden with publications on forensic pathology they had requested, I asked them why they had consulted me in particular. Baron's answer was what I would have guessed: none of the forensic pathologists in New York City would testify against Dr. Helpern, who was going to testify for the prosecution.

Although Baron seemed to think I was willing to rush in where angels feared to, the truth is I refuse an average of nine out of every ten cases I'm asked to get involved in. I consider myself courtroom-shy, and with good reason. As medical examiner, I heard witnesses I had interviewed—including policemen and detectives—give sworn testimony that bore little or no relation to what they had originally told me about criminal events and physical facts I remembered specifically and had officially recorded at the scene. On occasion, crucial documents or portions of police blotters relating to the case in point were missing and no longer available as evidence in court. And, on the witness stand, I have listened to rulings from the bench that were so arbitrary or irrational that I could only assume a "fix" or judicial cynicism.

I tend to wax philosophical about our judicial system. It has been said, "The expert sees only his learning, the judge sees only his court, and the jury sees humanity." Whoever said that was flattering most juries. Jury trials, our method of meting out justice, has been likened to a democracy, the worst system devised *except for all others.* I remember an eminent jurist once saying, "If I were accused of a crime and were innocent, I would ten thousand times take my chances with a jury rather than with the fairest and wisest judge who ever lived." "Ah, then," comes the reply, "And if you were guilty?"

The Crimmins case was obviously going to be won or lost on courtroom gamesmanship, and I wasn't sure I wanted to get involved in that. A little wrestling with myself made me see I was just being self-indulgent. The real issue was that Alice Crimmins had a right to the best defense possible. "It is better that nine and ninety guilty men should go free than one innocent man should be condemned." No matter how horrible our system is, it works.

My hang-ups resolved for the moment, I busied myself with an analysis of the autopsy findings on Alice Marie. The pertinent observations gleaned from the post-mortem description were these: numerous pinheadlike hemorrhages in the conjunctival lining of the lower eyelids and in the lining of the interior of the larynx (vocal box), smaller hemorrhages on the surfaces of the lungs and heart (these are all physical signs of asphyxia); and a small, poorly defined area of slight discoloration in the skin described as being at the angle formed by the left lower jaw with the neck and the lower portion of the ear. Except for this, the skin over the neck area was free of any changes. The skin here was intact, and there were no bruises, discolorations, or ligature marks. No hemorrhages, bruises, or lacerations were seen in the neck muscles. The larynx also contained no injury or fractures. The anus was relaxed, and the anal opening was somewhat dilated. The stomach contained partially digested food particles. Nothing else of significance was reported, and there was no mention of any microscopic examination of tissues removed at autopsy.

Martin Baron came alone to the next meeting and tried to extract from me anything I saw in the autopsy report that might conceivably favor his client's case. He pushed hard, but it was my obligation to resist any of his attempts to go beyond a fair and logical interpretation of the evidence. We explored all possibilities for challenges that might cast a reasonable doubt on the medical examiner's findings and conclusions. More specifically, we evaluated the strength of the evidence in support of strangulation as the cause of the asphyxia. Asphyxia literally means absence of the pulse, but as conventionally used by medical examiners, it means want of air and may be brought about by interference with the entrance of oxygen into the lungs. The oxygen can be prevented from entering the body by a block at the level of the nose and mouth; this is called suffocation. Mechanical interference in the region of the neck that hinders the passage of air through the main windpipe is called strangulation. Natural diseases in the lungs, such as pneumonia, allergies, and asthma, and in the throat, such as swelling from infections and croup, can also produce asphyxia. The diagnosis of asphyxia as the cause of death at autopsy can be exceedingly difficult. The so-called asphyxial picture present in Alice Marie, characterized by small hemorrhages, can also be simulated in natural disease. In the absence of microscopic study of the lungs, it was impossible for me to definitively exclude a naturally occurring illness.

The indictment of Alice Crimmins had specifically charged her with causing the death of her daughter by mechanical strangulation or ligature. Baron reasoned that, if the proof for strangulation as the cause of the asphyxia was inconclusive, it was plausible to suggest that the death might have been due to some other cause. He also speculated that grounds might then be established for an eventual appeal to the higher courts, were the outcome of the trial to result in a guilty verdict. I told him that, from the medical facts alone, the injuries seen at the autopsy were insufficient to determine the exact cause of the asphyxia, and this much I was willing to say in court. As for the significance of the partially digested food in the stomach, Baron, without giving me reasons, indicated he would rather stay away from this finding; I found out why during the second trial. Based upon the condition of the food particles in the stomach, the children had to have been fed at a certain time; this contradicted Mrs. Crimmins' testimony as to when she had fed them, jeopardizing her alibi.

He asked if the dilated anus could have been the result of sexual assault. It was a possibility, but asphyxia itself could also cause marked relaxation of the anus. Furthermore, there were no injuries in or around the anus to support a theory of forcible entry.

This case underscores what I have already said about pathologists specifically and now extend to all expert medical witnesses: The expert is not primarily involved with the ramifications of any case. He is not, and should not be, concerned with personalities, guilt, or innocence. His testimony must be prejudice free and within the limits of his area of training. How his interpretations relate to the other circumstances of the case is the province of the defense counsel. The lawyer tries to weave the expert's opinion into the entire fabric of his defense strategy. A case sometimes turns on a seemingly insignificant or unrelated technical detail. In this case, my review of the specifics of this autopsy revealed that there was no record of any microscopic sections. Microscopic lung sections could have been helpful in establishing a more definitive cause of death. The absence of these sections might be enough to shake the validity of the medical examiner's conclusions.

Homicide trials often need experts in such diverse fields as ballistics, X rays, chemistry, psychiatry, and pathology; without them, the defense, or even the prosecution, might have nothing to go on. Without them, countless cases could not be justly adjudicated. Some doctors participate in litigation only as undercover advisers; they work behind the scenes in the preparation of the legal brief and help frame questions for the cross-examination of the opposition witnesses. Many physicians do not relish coming into court, especially when they must face their counterparts testifying for the other side. Because two diverse "expert" opinions may be offered to the same jury, the practice of soliciting expert testimony has been criticized. The problem was succinctly commented upon many years ago by a judge in the New York Court of Appeals: "The fact has become very plain that in any case where opinion evidence is admissible, the particular kind of an opinion desired by any party to the controversy can be readily procured by paying the market price therefor." It has been claimed that some insurance companies have "stables of doctors" to say anything they want. Personal experience as an expert in cases of negligence, malpractice, workmen's compensation, double indemnity, and murder has made me suspicious of some members of my profession. A nationally known medical educator expressed it this way: "You get surprised at what people say in court; you never hear them say that in the medical societies or in the classroom."

Some lawyers advocate the elimination of this system, in which each side obtains and pays for its own experts, in favor of a system whereby the judge would have this authority. But many maintain that the present adversary process has a better-than-even chance of leading to the truth. I'm on the fence.

In preparing the opinion for attorneys Baron and Harrison, I found myself laboring under a handicap common to all medical consultants for the defense in a murder case: Our access to the medical information, and especially the autopsy, is always at second hand. We must rely upon the faithful recording of primary observations by others—the coroner's pathologist or the medical examiner—and assume these to be reliable and complete. Yet when one considers that Dr. Curran, Harvard's professor of forensic medicine, has estimated that less than 30 per cent of the United States is served by competent medical examiners, we have small reason to make such an assumption. This means that first crack at 70 per cent of homicide autopsies is in the hands of relative incompetents. I have found, too often, glaring errors or omissions in the original examination when I have done reautopsies.

Here, in the Crimmins case, I had to accept Dr. Helpern's findings at face value. I will willingly grant that he is a talented, highly competent practitioner. But even the best among us has his bad days, when a bit of carelessness or an oversight goes undetected. My most embarrassing mistake occurred in a workmen's compensation case: The man had died of a heart attack, and in my autopsy report I had incidentally described two normal kidneys. During the hearing, X rays were introduced that showed the man had had one kidney removed. Although the finding had no bearing on the case, my credibility and competence were a bit diminished by the mistake. How did it happen? I'd autopsied the man on a particularly harried Sunday, along with seven other urgent autopsies. In transcribing my findings at the end of the day, I neglected to record my observation of the missing kidney. Being rushed is no excuse for a mistake, but it explains how a lot of innocent blunders are allowed to distort conclusions.

District attorneys are aware of their experts' advantage at having primary access to a body and are sure to use it as a weapon during trial. The district attorney, on cross-examination of the defense expert, will ask the source of information. He usually asks in such a way—as did the district attorney of me in the Crimmins case—as to imply that the information is distorted because it is secondhand.

But the defense expert has an advantage over the prosecution that counterbalances this tactic: hindsight. Since his examination occurs after other evidence has been accumulated, he has the tools and the time to seek out any errors or deficiencies in the conduct and the findings of the post-mortem examination. The medical examiner is stuck with his original report; if he discovers an error at a later date and corrects it (which a disconcerting number of medical examiners don't), he opens himself to a suspicion of incompetence. Having been a medical examiner myself, I know that it is impossible to anticipate every twist of a given case. The only safeguard is to perform the most complete and accurate autopsy possible, not to omit any of the routine basic tests on the blood, tissues, or gastric contents, and to record the findings accurately and in complete detail.

The medical examiner has a more sacred duty than serving the needs of the prosecutor. He has to be doubly sure that the case is actually a homicide. Failure to be scrupulous in this regard has resulted in the unjust conviction and punishment of many innocent persons. And in the Crimmins case, a serious question did exist as to whether there was proof beyond any reasonable doubt that Alice Marie's death was an unnatural one. Dr. Richard Grimes, of Helpern's own department, and first at the scene, had serious misgivings about this and expressed these

doubts at the trial. At that time, Grimes had retired and was
no longer under Helpern's authority.

A case in point was one I had as a neophyte medical examiner in Westchester County. It began with the relatively commonplace occurrence of a tired housewife and mother of a
couple of children getting into an argument with her drunken
husband. He had arrived home in his usual, intoxicated state.
Exasperated with his behavior, she threw a plate, which hit him
in the forehead. The next morning, he awoke with a slight headache. During the day it worsened, and, when he reached a
nearby hospital, his condition was considered serious enough to
require admission. By that afternoon, he was comatose, and he
died a few hours later, before a diagnosis could be made. The
hospital authorities notified the police, the county district attorney, and the medical examiner's office. The district attorney prepared a preliminary warrant for the woman's arrest on a homicide charge but held it in abeyance until he heard from me. I examined the husband's body and found an extensive hemorrhage
and blood clots beneath the membranes covering the brain. I
searched for the source of the bleeding. After carefully cleaning
off most of the blood clot from the surface of the brain, and
after a tedious dissection of the narrow and fragile blood vessels
feeding into the brain's undersurface, I located a tiny, tissue-
paper-thin sac, less than one quarter of an inch in diameter,
bulging from one of these small-caliber arteries. It contained
a small perforation from which the blood had leaked, covering
and compressing the entire brain. The technical name for this
condition is an "aneurysm of a cerebral blood vessel." This kind
of defect is a naturally occurring abnormality, and rupture of
it occurs as a spontaneous event entirely unrelated to any external injury or physical force. This was the cause of death, and
the plate-throwing episode was a strange coincidence that had
no bearing on the cerebral hemorrhage. Upon notification of

my final diagnosis, the district attorney, for once enthusiastically, suspended any further legal action against the wife.

Analogous cases with coincidental violence in which there has either been no autopsy or only a cursory or incompetent dissection of the body have been incorrectly reported as homicides to district attorneys across the country.

With all of this roiling in my mind the night before I was to testify in the Alice Crimmins case, I became anxious, a feeling I hadn't encountered in other trial situations. I have always had some apprehension before appearing in court and have usually experienced some slight pretrial nervousness, but this was different. I knew Mrs. Crimmins was to follow me on the stand as soon as I finished testifying. Her appearance guaranteed that the barnlike courtroom, with a seating capacity of five hundred, would be filled. The newspapers had predicted long lines of people waiting to get in. The anticipated circus-like atmosphere superimposed on an already troubling situation—a woman's life hanging in the balance—most likely provoked my excessive anxiety.

This courtroom game was being played for a woman's life. The players were the accused, Alice Crimmins; the prosecutor, District Attorney Mosley; the main defense counsel, Martin Baron; the judge, Peter T. Farrell; and an all-male jury. Each of the two camps observed the accepted rules of restraint. But at a certain critical point in the course of this bizarre game, the antagonisms accelerate. There is no clear before or after, but imperceptibly, as the trial nears its end, it reaches the dangerous zone, where the defendant is condemned to win or lose all: guilty, with the possibility of life internment, or not guilty, with freedom to begin a new life. And in the Alice Crimmins case my anxiety was heightened by the possibility that this dangerous point of no return might arrive while I was still on the stand.

On May 22, I was called as the first witness for the defense in the afternoon session of the court. As I recall, Martin Baron began his direct examination by asking me when I graduated from medical school and became licensed to practice medicine in the state of New York. My answer was: "In 1936."

Q. "Do you practice any medical specialty?"

A. "Yes, pathology."

Q. "What is a pathologist?"

A. "A pathologist is a physician who specializes in studying the changes in the tissues of the body caused by disease or injury. Among his functions is the performance of autopsies. Pathology has legal, diagnostic, research, and teaching aspects. Over the years, I have engaged in all four of these functions."

Q. "How many autopsies have you performed or supervised during your career as a pathologist?"

A. "Well over ten thousand."

Q. "What has been your experience and training as a pathologist?" (At this point, I enumerated all my experiences and positions in hospitals and teaching positions in medical schools, as well as my research appointments.)

Q. "Have you ever served as a medical examiner?"

A. "Yes, I was chief medical examiner of Westchester County from 1949 to 1953 and was in charge of the forensic medicine course for many years at Columbia University."

Q. "Have you had an opportunity to examine the autopsy report on the deceased Alice Marie?"

A. "Yes, I have."

Q. "Do you have an opinion as to the cause of death?"

A. "Yes, I do."

Q. "What is your opinion?"

A. "I believe Alice Marie died from asphyxia, which means insufficient oxygen in the body."

Q. "Do you have an opinion as to the cause of the asphyxia?"

A. "Based on the limited autopsy report, which does not include microscopic examination of the tissues, I can only speculate as to the cause for the asphyxia. It may have been due to suffocation, possibly to strangulation, and possibly due to other, natural diseases."

Q. "Are you able to state beyond any reasonable doubt that the asphyxia was caused by strangulation?"

A. "No, I cannot, because the autopsy report does not mention any significant injuries to the skin and muscles of the neck or to the windpipe. In order to be more certain about strangulation as the cause, some of these areas should show evidence of injury."

Q. "Is there any evidence that Alice Marie may have been sexually assaulted?"

A. "The only suggestion in the autopsy report was a dilated anus, but this could just as well have been caused by the asphyxia."

Q. "Can you absolutely exclude natural causes for the asphyxia?"

A. "No, I cannot."

This, in essence, concluded the questioning by Martin Baron. District Attorney Mosley began his cross-examination. He is a tall, powerful, well-built man with a manner of asking questions that could easily intimidate an inexperienced witness. Although the cross-examination took close to two hours, there were only a few questions really pertinent to the case. Most of the preliminary questions can be classified as diversionary. To the best of my recollection, it was as follows:

Q. "Dr. Spain, are you personally acquainted with the defendant?"

A. "No, I have never met or spoken to the defendant."

Q. "Are you receiving a fee for your testimony?"

A. "I am receiving the customary fee for the time spent in consultation with the defendant's attorneys and for the time required for me to be present in court."

Q. "What was the source of your information, upon which you based your opinion as to the cause of death?"

A. "On a copy of the medical examiner's description of the autopsy."

Q. "That is all?"

A. "Yes."

Q. "In other words, you did not directly participate in or personally attend the autopsy yourself, and otherwise have no new first-hand facts on which you base your opinion?"

A. "No, I do not."

Q. "Are you acquainted with Dr. Milton Helpern?"

A. "Yes, we worked side by side in the Bellevue autopsy room for almost ten years and have been professional colleagues appearing in situations together since that time."

Q. "Are you familiar with his work and his reputation?"

A. "Yes."

Q. "Is he regarded as an authority in the field?"

A. "Yes."

(All these questions were of course designed to diminish the value of my opinion in relation to that of Dr. Helpern's.)

Q. "You are familiar with Dr. Helpern's conclusions that strangulation was the cause of the asphyxia?"

A. "Yes, I am."

Q. "And you disagree with it?"

A. "Yes, I disagree with it in the sense that other possibilities have not been completely excluded."

Q. "What other possibilities?"

A. "Suffocation and natural death."

At this point, District Attorney Mosley cited portions of Dr. Helpern's testimony and asked if I disagreed or agreed.

A. "I think all I can say is that there was asphyxia possibly caused by strangulation, smothering, or other existing things. Dr. Helpern's autopsy report is incomplete because it does not include microscopic tissue examination."

The district attorney then approached the bench. He asked for a temporary recess to permit me to read portions of Dr. Helpern's testimony at this trial describing the microscopic findings omitted from the original and only autopsy report. The slides had never been submitted into evidence. This precluded any opportunity for the defense to requisition them for my examination, and I was forced to rely entirely on Dr. Helpern's opinion. After reading this material I returned to the stand, and District Attorney Mosley continued his cross-examination:

Q. "Has the reading of this testimony and Dr. Helpern's opinion on the slides in any way altered your previous opinion as to the cause of the asphyxia, and do you still disagree with Dr. Helpern's conclusions in this case?"

A. "There was nothing in his testimony to make me modify my already stated views."

Besides giving testimony that was damaging to Mr. Baron's case, Dr. Helpern had also given some testimony that should have helped it considerably. Mr. Baron on cross-examination got Dr. Helpern to confirm that Dr. Luke, a medical examiner in his department, under his supervision, had published, with his approval, an article in the January 1967 issue of *The Archives of Pathology* unequivocally stating that in the experiences with strangulation of the New York City medical examiner's office "there are no confirmed cases of manual strangulation in the group without external neck injury." If the jury had been alert and attentive, this should have created serious misgivings. Alice Crimmins was charged with strangulation, and the only neck injury Dr. Grimes had reported was an area of slight discoloration near the lower ear.

District Attorney Mosley's final question was:

Q. "Did you have any discussions or conferences with anyone concerning your testimony and other matters relating to this case?"

A. "Yes, I had two meetings in my office with the defense attorneys and several telephone discussions with them. I had no other conferences or dialogue with anyone else."

The district attorney's question was designed to create a suspicion that there might have been something not quite aboveboard about our meetings.

Martin Baron had no questions for me on redirect examination, and I was excused as a witness.

The New York *Times* reported that during my description of the clinical details of Alice Marie's body (or Missy, as they called her), Alice Crimmins kept her eyes downcast. When I was finally excused, she took the stand in her own defense and began to testify in a whisper. When the judge repeatedly asked her to respond more loudly, she became speechless and was led weeping from the stand. A recess was declared until 10:00 A.M. the next day.

Until my court appearance was reported in the press, only a few close friends had known of my connection with this case. When my involvement became public knowledge, neighbors, friends, and a few relatives became instant experts on my motives for testifying on behalf of Alice Crimmins and had much to say about it: "He must be doing it for the publicity." "I'll bet he's getting a real fat fee for helping to get her off the hook." "I just don't understand him. How could he permit his name to be linked with someone obviously guilty?" "I could understand it if this were a political case, but what has Alice Crimmins got to do with the civil-rights movement?" Finally, one sympathetic comment: "Dr. Spain always testifies for the underdog."

None of these people understood the essential role of the expert witness in our adversary system of justice. Most had judged this case long before the defense had produced its first witness. And how could the public think differently? From the time of the indictment until the trial in May, the news media had been filled with sensational stories about Alice Crimmins' personal life, all rife with innuendos of numerous extramarital romantic relationships and the neglect of her children. All that was left was to pronounce the sentence.

It remained for a long-time acquaintance to confront me with the ugliest comment. "How could you, a respectable and well-regarded pathologist, permit your knowledge and reputation to be used on behalf of this Irish whore who murdered her own children?" My response was instantaneous. "Would it be all right with you if she were a Jewish whore?" My friend was completely unprepared for my sarcasm, but I believe he got the point. To my surprise, men more than women reacted with hostility at the mere mention of Mrs. Crimmins' name.

It was easy to get a distorted impression of my testimony from the reports in the newspapers. Unless a reader was well versed in how they twist the facts, he could easily believe I had sworn under oath that little Alice Marie had died from natural causes and that this was no homicide. But this misconception was not as important as the failure of most people to comprehend the basic tenet of our system of criminal justice: any person, man, woman, black, yellow, or white, Jew or Christian, alcoholic or teetotaler, prude or whore, is presumed to be innocent of a crime until proven guilty beyond any reasonable doubt. They could not concede that this woman, fighting for her life, was entitled to at least the same quality of help and expertise in her defense as was so abundantly and readily available to the district attorney, who had all the resources of the state's law-enforcement agencies at his disposal.

When I realized that my friends had already decided on Mrs. Crimmins' guilt because of her personal life, I realized the impossibility of selecting a truly unbiased and fair-minded jury. I answered most of the comments concerning my role in the trial by saying, "Why go through the charade of a trial? Why not get it over with and just hang Alice Crimmins from a tree?"

Mrs. Crimmins was judged guilty in the slaying of her daughter and was sentenced to from five to twenty-five years in prison. With good behavior she would have been free in five years. She was a young woman; there was still time to start a new life. But she was stubbornly determined to prove her innocence and insisted that Martin Baron conduct a vigorous appeal.

Rumors had reached the ears of Baron about an illegal act committed during the course of the trial by some of the jurors. Persistent interrogation of these men finally yielded pay dirt: Baron uncovered the fact that three of the jurors had made a secret, unauthorized visit to the scene of the alleged crime before reaching a final decision in the case. This unorthodox act, an unquestionable violation of ethical jurors' behavior, forced the state court of appeals to void the guilty verdict, declare a mistrial, and order a new trial.

Alice Crimmins was released on bail and was again technically presumed innocent until proven guilty. This was the immediate, practical result of Baron's exposé.

But he came across something else during his investigation that really rocked me: "The twelve men who sat as jurors during the first trial hated Alice Crimmins." Theirs was no dispassionate decision. They detested her. The district attorney, aware that men are capable of greater hostility in a jury situation than women, had exploited this tendency by using his challenges effectively to keep all women off this jury. Obviously, then, without women this was in no sense a jury of Alice Crimmins' peers.

In the second trial, Alice Crimmins was unexpectedly confronted with the additional charge of the first-degree murder of Edmund, Jr. This belated indictment was not only vindictive, but had seemed legally precluded, because the medical examiner had been unable to prove a cause of death and did not list the death as a homicide. In the years following, nothing new was discovered to alter Dr. Helpern's earlier opinion. The legal basis for the new indictment rested upon a little-known, flimsy, and rarely used legal precedent: in instances in which more than one corpse is found within the context of the same suspected crime, the determination of homicide in one of the victims may be used to assume the same in the second body when conditions have hindered proving the cause of death.

Alice Crimmins was again judged guilty, but this time for the murder of both children. Because of the additional conviction on the first-degree murder charge, she received a mandatory sentence of life imprisonment. Of great influence on the outcome of the second trial was Dr. Helpern's opinion on the probable time of death and the likely time the children had their last meal. His determination was based on the degree of digestion of the food particles found in Alice Marie's stomach at autopsy. On this, Dr. Helpern stood firm about the validity of this evidence. He was correct in doing so, but I could not help remembering that Friday afternoon in his office, when we met to resolve our differences in the Tombs suicide case. At that time, he was presented with similar evidence in the form of gastric contents, observed and described by his own protégé, Dr. Baden. Then Dr. Helpern had hemmed and hawed when asked for his opinion, and in effect had responded, "One cannot be certain in these matters." Now, only a short time later, in the second trial of Alice Crimmins, his testimony on the meaning of the gastric contents was crucial. Some legal buffs believed this was one of the decisive factors leading to a guilty verdict.

It is ironic that Alice Crimmins' life sentence arose from her insistence, after the initial conviction, on proving her innocence. Had the higher court rejected her appeal, she would not have been faced with a second charge of murder. At the moment, five years of her sentence have already passed. She would now have been eligible for release on good behavior.

Guilty or not, she was the object of hate from a jury blinded by contempt and hostility and was the real-life victim of a trial not unlike that depicted in Lewis Carroll's *Alice's Adventures in Wonderland.* "Sentence first, verdict afterwards."

Baron was not the attorney in the second trial, but the new one had called to ask if I could possibly be of help to him in the defense. I refrained from becoming involved, because, after reviewing the evidence as it unfolded in the first trial, I realized my testimony had been of little or no value in influencing the course of the case. I had no reason to believe that it would be any different in the second trial.

By the time the first trial had run its course, I had formed my own opinion concerning Alice Crimmins' guilt or innocence. But my opinion didn't matter; it was and is irrelevant to the entire situation and the issues of my concern.

The saddest part of all is that the jury and the adversary system of justice is the best that man has yet been able to devise.

Alice Crimmins spent two years in jail while her case was appealed. Finally, on May 7, 1973, the Appellate Division of the New York State Supreme Court ruled on her case and reversed both the murder and the manslaughter convictions in the deaths of her two children. The five judges unanimously dismissed the murder conviction involving the death of her son, Edmund, Jr. In a three-to-two decision they also ruled that she was entitled to a new trial on the manslaughter charge of killing her daughter, Alice Marie. With respect to the first opinion the judges said, "we believe the corpus delicti [cause of death] was not established since as a matter of law the people did not prove beyond a reasonable doubt that his death [Edmund, Jr.'s] resulted from a criminal act." In the second reversal the Appellate Division stated that the prosecutor's summation was "grossly improper and prejudicial" and also that the trial judge, Queens Supreme Court Justice George V. Balbach, committed several prejudicial errors.

Aside from the meaning of this to Alice Crimmins (who was first arrested on September 12, 1967), I felt gratified that my previous uneasiness about the outcome of this case was substantiated by the higher court's decision. I fully concur with the sentiments expressed by New York *Post* columnist Pete Hamill: "But there has been enough punishment now. Enough. Alice Crimmins has lived eight tortured years. She will never get them back. Her life will never again be what it was before that humid July morning long ago. It's time for some mercy."

2. ABORTION AND THE BATTERED CHILD

I am the only being whose doom
No tongue would ask, no eye would mourn.
I never caused a thought of gloom,
A smile of joy, since I was born.

Emily Brontë, I AM THE ONLY BEING

My mother groan'd! my father wept.
Into the dangerous world I lept:
Helpless, naked, piping loud:
Like a fiend hid in a cloud.

William Blake, INFANT SORROW

To many people, the most important question in the current controversy is whether or not abortion constitutes the taking of a life. That was the important question for me, too, for quite a while. I firmly believed that a doctor had no right to play God and decide when to terminate life. I was categorically opposed to abortion, euthanasia, and suicide. My role was to prolong life, no matter what, even if the patient was dying and in the throes of an agonizing last seizure.

A lot of things happened to shake my conception of the doctor's role. The first was in my first year as medical examiner of Westchester County. A county parkway-police officer on patrol came across a large mongrel dog with what looked like an animal body dangling from its mouth. He chased the dog, and the dog dropped the bundle it was carrying. It turned out to be the partially decomposed body of a very small infant. The officer brought the body to my laboratory for identification.

We autopsied the body and found it to be a human fetus of about six months' development. The wooded area where the officer had seen the dog was searched. A clearing nearby was found to contain many more of these small, decomposing bodies. Some were strewn on the surface of the clearing, and others were partially buried. They varied in age, but most were almost fully mature fetuses. A rambling frame house close by contained enough suggestive equipment to mark it as an abandoned abortion factory. Its operators were never caught.

The number of bodies staggered me, but they represented a tiny fraction of illegal abortions performed annually in this country. It was estimated that in New York State alone, one hundred thousand a year were performed illegally. Obviously, not that many ever came to light; only where there are complications, or death, do abortions come to public attention.

My next experience came in the form of a small bundle wrapped in one of our department's new, economical, disposable paper shrouds. Jim Florence had responded to a call from the police to pick up the body of a dead baby in White Plains. As I was unwrapping the body, I noticed the tag attached. It said: CHARLES THOMAS.* It hit me very hard; this had been a baby boy.

Charles Thomas was a sickening sight. The body was emaci-

* All the names in this chapter are pseudonyms, but otherwise the cases are real.

ated, the eyes set in a face that was little more than a skull, a head too large for the shrunken, wrinkled body. The belly was swollen. The whole carcass was covered with crawling maggots.

We did some investigating after this horror-movie episode and discovered that Charles Thomas had been willfully neglected by his parents. He was the product of an accidental conception. After his birth, his parents carefully refrained from feeding him. They didn't want him around. He was about a month old when he died. At a hearing, the parents were put under custody of the family court, and their other child was placed in a residential treatment center.

This was an obvious case. There are more subtle examples of child battering and child neglect, as I discovered when a lawyer for legal aid called me about a consultation regarding the death of a four-month-old male baby. He wasn't defending the child's parents; his client was an eleven-year-old boy who had been babysitting for the victim the night the dead baby was found. I asked the attorney to mail me a copy of the autopsy report in advance of our meeting; my experience with legal-aid lawyers has been that they tend to procrastinate, usually for reasons of overwork. I was delighted when the report arrived the next morning. As it turned out, this lawyer had given the case considerable thought and was meticulous in gathering the essential facts.

The pertinent facts in the autopsy on the male baby, Alfred Dexter, performed by an assistant medical examiner in a large urban center, were as follows:

". . . a linear crusted area over the right frontal region [forehead] measuring 1 x ⅛ inches
. . . over the right cheek are two lines of small ovoid, purplish red contused areas, separated by a clear space—the two together

form a teeth biting pattern; individual tooth marked area measured $\frac{3}{16}$ inch in greatest diameter, intervening space of 1 inch.
. . . extensive hemorrhage in the diaphragm.
. . . contused areas posteriorly [back] in both lungs and immediately adjacent to hilum [roots of lung].
. . . The dome of the liver is almost bisected by a large gaping
laceration [tear] measuring 4 inches [other lacerations were
also described].
. . . The surface of the liver shows extensive subcapsular hemorrhage
. . . 300 cc. of blood in abdominal cavity."

Then followed the conclusions: "I hereby certify that on the
24th day of November, 1966, I made an autopsy of the body
of Alfred Dexter now lying dead at the General Hospital Mortuary and upon investigation of the essential facts concerning
the circumstances of the death and history of the case, I am of
the opinion that the cause of death was:

1. Lacerations of liver, with contusions of lung and diaphragm
2. Massive intraperitoneal hemorrhage
3. Homicidal."

The medical examiner in charge of this case did not express
any doubts as to his verdict and unequivocally stated that the
baby died as a result of the torn liver and hemorrhagic injuries.
As far as he was concerned, it was a homicide.

A first superficial reading of this report, especially in the absence of any background information, led me to concur with this
official interpretation. But somehow I was left with an uneasy
feeling about the medical examiner's conclusion. When the
counsel from the legal aid society arrived for a conference, I
learned that Kenneth, cousin of the slain baby, had been charged
with homicide and was now in the custody of the family court.

The evening of the death, Kenneth had been hired as the babysitter for the Dexters. They had two sons: Alfred, four months old, and David, two and one half years of age. The Dexters were away from the apartment three hours. Upon their return, they found Kenneth sound asleep, sprawled out on the sofa with the television set on. In the bedroom both of their sons seemed asleep; Alfred, the baby, was on the large double bed, and David was on the floor next to his toys. Mr. Dexter lifted the baby to place him in his crib. As he did, he noted that Alfred was not breathing and that the body appeared unusually limp. He called to his wife and then rushed to the phone and called for an ambulance. They awakened Kenneth and asked him what had happened. He claimed not to know what they were talking about. The ambulance arrived and rushed the infant to the hospital, where he was pronounced dead upon arrival.

An autopsy was performed by the local medical examiner's office. When the autopsy findings were revealed, Kenneth became the main suspect. Repeated and lengthy interrogation of Kenneth by the detectives and investigators from the DA's office failed to gain an admission of assault on Alfred. His account of the evening was simple and straightforward. According to him, after the Dexters left the apartment the baby and the little boy were quiet, so he went into the living room and watched television. Once he thought he heard some whimpering coming from the bedroom. He looked in. The baby was asleep, and David was on the floor playing with a fire engine. His next recollection was being awakened by the Dexters.

Independent examinations of Kenneth by a court-assigned psychiatrist and child psychologist uncovered nothing to indicate a behavioral disorder or psychopathic sexual tendencies. His teachers said he was co-operative in class, was a moderately good student, and had many friends. Nevertheless the homicide charge stuck, probably because nothing was found to incriminate anyone else. The DA also wanted to get the irate parents off his neck.

The legal-aid lawyer's story reinforced the persistent nagging doubt I had about the soundness of the medical examiner's interpretation of the autopsy findings. I had an intuitive feeling that Kenneth was entirely innocent of any wrongdoing in this affair. But why? Even conceding for the moment that Alfred's death was caused by a physical assault, the unlikely combination of a small human bite on the baby's cheek and the much grosser fatal physical damage to the liver did not ring true. While I was mulling over this incongruity in my mind, the lawyer, as if sensing my thoughts, asked if it were a physical possibility for the two-and-one-half-year-old brother of the deceased to have inflicted the fatal injuries. He hastened to add that the relatively large size of the bite on the cheek seemed to eliminate the little brother because of the discrepancy between the small size of his mouth and that of the actual bite. These last remarks sparked something in me. There was an obvious technical point about the bite mark I should have considered during my first reading of the autopsy. I, too, was misled by its size. I should have realized that bites on soft tissue with loose overlying skin, such as the cheek, pull the skin together into a fold, between the two rows of teeth. Upon release of the bite the margins retract and the upper and lower teeth marks would now have a wider space between them than at the time of the bite. These bite marks could, then, have been produced by the smaller mouth of David. I simulated the situation and made appropriate measurements. These tended to support my revised view of the situation, even though I was aware of my inexperience in the field of bite analysis. It did lead me to the discovery that there had been an amazing oversight in the forensic pathological investigation of this case. No one had bothered to check if the suspect's dentition matched the bite marks on Alfred's cheek.

Nor had the bite been excised and kept as permanent evidence. Perhaps the medical examiner, attaching little or no significance to it, did not wish to disfigure the face. Unfortunately, he also neglected to photograph it. He did, however, record the markings in some detail in his report.

Mainly to strengthen Kenneth's defense, the lawyer, at my suggestion, called in a dental expert; he made an impression of the suspect's dentition and compared it with a reconstructed version of the bite marks. They did not match. The next logical step would have been to do the same with David, but we dared not approach the parents on this. I am sure that if it had become a crucial point we could have insisted on it.

Bite-mark investigation is an entrancing but difficult undertaking, because most marks never reproduce accurately the dental features of the originator. For one thing, they usually include only a very limited number of teeth, and, secondly, the human skin in which the mark has been left is a poor impression material, with varying qualities of shrinkage and distortion. In Kenneth's case, however, the discrepancies between his dentition and the bite were so great that there was little doubt that he was not the cause of the bite. But, after all, the bite was not the injury that caused death, and it could have been inflicted on another occasion by David. The finding was sufficient, nevertheless, to raise my index of doubt, which led to the next question, that of the injuries to the liver, lungs, and diaphragm. My initially uncritical acceptance of the medical examiner's interpretation of the cause of death had dulled my curiosity to the extent that I had failed to consider another possibility. I hadn't asked an essential question. No one, not the medical examiner, the district attorney's man, the detectives, or even the defense attorney, had exhibited any interest in knowing if any mechanical method of resuscitation had been applied to Alfred's body in the ambulance while en route to the hospital. I suddenly became so anxious to get at this information that I must have sounded incoherent when I asked the lawyer if he had any copies of the ambulance and emergency-room treatment reports. He wasn't sure, but he delved into his briefcase and pulled out a bundle of papers. Thumbing through them, he found these records. He happened to have them only because he was an obsessively meticulous attorney. He never really considered that they might have some bearing on the case, and there was no reason why he should have thought so. At the moment I asked the question, I felt certain of the answer. Yes! Alfred had received mechanical resuscitation for at least fifteen minutes while in the ambulance.

I had anticipated the attorney's response, because, like many other pathologists, I have in recent years seen this pattern: injuries as the result of trauma from the overzealous and too forceful application of mechanical resuscitation and external cardiac massage. This occurs more frequently in younger patients, where the chest wall is still quite fragile and tissues easily torn. These injuries are regarded as artifacts usually occurring after death; they do not in any way contribute to the death of the individual. So in Alfred's case, this could now be dismissed as the likely cause of his demise. The injuries were only a consequence of the heroic efforts to revive him. Nothing is absolute, but the chances that the injuries killed him were now considered slight.

Fortified with this new information, plus the question marks relating to the timing and origin of the cheek bite, we were encouraged to speculate on alternative theories concerning the manner and cause of Alfred's death. This time, for a fleeting moment, I did feel a kinship with Perry Mason, who not only always vindicates his clients but simultaneously finds the real killers.

Because the bite mark closely coincided with the size of

David's mouth, I postulated that the two-and-one-half-year-old brother could have climbed astride the baby, bitten him on the cheek and accidentally smothered him. Or else he could have playfully bounced up and down on Alfred and caused serious damage to his internal organs. This could have been playful, or subconsciously the result of sibling jealousy, not uncommon in children of David's age with similar circumstances of a new intruder into the family. It was a reasonable series of speculations. But it was incapable of proof or disproof. To interrogate the little boy, who could at best mumble one or two words, would have been cruel and useless.

More likely, Alfred's death was entirely spontaneous and natural, from a mysterious cause popularly referred to as "crib death." This poorly understood condition exacts a toll of about twenty-five thousand sudden and unexpected deaths in apparently healthy young babies each year in this country alone. And it has been in the attempts at revival of these cases that I have seen much of the damage caused by resuscitative techniques. Here again, there was no way of being absolutely certain.

Once Kenneth seemed to be in the clear—the alternative theories had been successful in having the charges reconsidered—I had time to relax and look a bit more deeply into the parents' role in the whole affair. In the back of my mind, I still thought: "battered child." I had just received a report of the Department of Health alerting physicians to the increasing frequency of these brutalities, which do not always result in death. I had seen such a child, covered with bruises, a broken bone or two, a small human standing half dazed, in pain, frightened and helpless, with little or no comprehension of what had befallen him or why. It can never be eradicated from one's sensibilities. The child is surrounded by the impersonal hospital emergency room. The police photographer, in a cold, routine, businesslike way, is shooting pictures of the child from every angle, to capture the details of each injury. The doctor is poking around to get his job done, and the nurse, detective, or social worker is plying the child with an endless series of questions. The little person, in his innocence, thinks this befell him because he did something bad; then he begins to believe he really was bad. Not understanding he is an unwanted child, his only desire is to be held, and smothered with tenderness.

Common behavioral patterns that lead one to suspect parents of neglect or physical abuse of a child include weak explanatory tales at variance with the clinical findings; reluctance on their part to give any information; delay in seeking medical help; inappropriate reactions by them relative to the severity of the injuries to the child; and their tendency to place the blame for the abuse upon a third party.

The Dexters had committed four acts that evening which bothered me: A crib was present in the room, yet they departed leaving the helpless baby lying unprotected on a wide-open double bed from which he could have rolled off. They had asked Kenneth to come over only a few minutes before they went out for the evening. As far as I could learn, they were unusually calm when the ambulance arrived. Lastly was the haste with which they pointed the finger at Kenneth.

Did they leave the house knowing the baby was already dead either from an accidental fall from the bed or from a blow that one of them had struck in a fit of anger? Did one of them drop the baby and put it back on the bed, not aware that a fatal injury had already been inflicted? But, in all these conjectures, I came up against a stalemate of my own making. If my interpretation of the injuries—which we hoped would absolve Kenneth—was correct, I could not now make an about-face and reinterpret these same injuries as having been incurred before death in order to point the finger at the parents. Confronted with this dilemma, we realized nothing more could come of our deliberations. The lawyer and I decided to call a halt.

The attorney, using material from our discussion, prepared a legal brief outlining Kenneth's defense. When he presented this at the pretrial hearing in the family court, the judge decided the district attorney had failed to establish a prima facie case against Kenneth. He dismissed the charges. No further light was ever shed on the mystery of Alfred's death.

Of all the possible explanations for Alfred's death, I suppose I favored most "crib death." In cases like that of the Dexters, one is hard put to decide whether an infant's death is the genuine phenomenon of crib death or whether it is a result of mistreatment. Crib deaths occur suddenly and unexpectedly, and are spontaneous: no human agent causes them. The deaths occur in apparently healthy young babies, without any prior warning, usually at about the age of two months. The infants are found dead in their cribs, cots, or carriages. Despite a continuing research effort and the annual introduction of new concepts and theories, little more is known about these crib deaths than bare statistics. The core of the problem remains unpenetrated.

A young couple who had suffered the loss of a three-month-old daughter from crib death came to me for reassurance and some sort of insight into the enigma. I had performed the autopsy on the Webers' baby. Underlying their questions was the need to understand the nature and cause of their child's death. Equally relevant were two other questions: Had the Webers themselves or had the infant's pediatrician been negligent in any manner whatsoever that could account for the fatality, and could it have been prevented? If in the future another child was to be born to them, what was the risk of history repeating itself? I had been asked these questions many times before by parents under similar circumstances, and the answers were on the tip of my tongue. Actually I had prepared a form letter that was automatically mailed to all such parents explaining in simple language all that was currently known about this problem. They always came to my office anyway, for further and more personal reassurance.

The Webers were told that the best medical evidence to date did not reveal any genetic, inheritable, or family tendencies for crib deaths. I, in a sense, gave them a guarantee that in the event of another child, the chance for the same thing happening again would be most unlikely, and the risk would be no greater than in a family in which this had never occurred. To relieve them of any guilt feelings in themselves, or concern over the reliability of their pediatrician, I tried to convince them there was not the slightest indication of any carelessness or wrongdoing on their or the doctor's part. I repeatedly emphasized that the decisive gap in our knowledge about the cause did not detract from the fact they could have more children with impunity.

Because I was doing a study of this subject, I probed into Mrs. Weber's past medical history and uncovered that, years before the birth of this baby, she had had an illegal abortion. It was improperly performed, and an infection developed. It took many years of medical and surgical treatment before she could become pregnant again. Not directly related to my study, but because the entire question of the ethics and morality of abortion had been plaguing me for some time, I asked her why she had had the abortion and how she felt about abortions now, since she had had such a difficult time getting pregnant again, after the tragic loss of her only child. Her response was totally unexpected. Mr. and Mrs. Weber had decided in favor of the abortion together. It was during the Korean War, and there was a period when the threat of atomic warfare was a conceivable and immediate reality. They had been married for a short period, and their future was uncertain. As Mrs. Weber said, "I didn't want to bring a child into this world with the

threat of extinction hanging over its head. Also, both of us were
not emotionally prepared for another member in the family."
Mr. Weber added: "If abortions had been legal at that time,
there would have been no infection and my wife wouldn't have
had the difficulties she had in becoming pregnant again." They
both agreed that, despite the death of their baby, whether or
not one should have an abortion should be a personal decision.

Their desire, in face of their hardships, to see a child brought
into the right physical and emotional environment helped me
to see that doctors should be concerned not only with life itself;
they must also consider the personal quality of life and have
an active concern with the quality of the external environment
into which a life is being born.

Actually seeing what lengths women would go to, what they
would do to themselves in order to excise the "intruder," finally
made me realize that women's reproductive systems have been
enslaved by existing anti-abortion laws. I performed an autopsy
on a young woman I will call Joan G.

Late one evening, she had been rushed into a Mt. Vernon
hospital in a semicoma. The emergency-room physician could
obtain only a useless, fragmentary history of her illness from
her parents. They knew she had been well until six days before.
Then, one morning, she stayed home from her secretarial job
at a high school because she felt feverish and had an intense
headache. She would not permit her parents to call a physician.
Her condition rapidly worsened. When she could no longer respond to them, her parents called their family doctor. He took
one look and called for an ambulance, and a few hours after admission to the hospital, she died. No diagnosis had been
established. Because of the lack of any concrete information
surrounding the circumstances of her acute illness, and with no
proven cause of death, the case was reported to the medical
examiner's office.

At the autopsy I found the remains of a recently performed incomplete abortion. There was a perforation in the vault of her vagina, and her abdominal cavity was filled with pus. She had a fulminating peritonitis. A long knitting needle was protruding from the hole in her vagina into the abdominal cavity. This improvised tool had carried the bacteria into her body; the fatality was the result of an amateurish abortion attempt.

Whether this was a "do it yourself" job, or whether Joan had fallen into the hands of some irresponsible individual, was never determined. It is a reasonable supposition that Joan, unable to confide in anyone she felt would understand or anyone she could trust, was driven to this desperate act by an ancient law and outmoded code of morality that prevented her from openly and legally obtaining proper advice and help.

If the butchery had indeed been performed by an abortionist, Joan had probably been led to him by friends in a similar predicament. It may have been her desire to protect them that kept her from telling her parents and in refusing the services of a doctor. This made it impossible for anyone to recognize the complications and denied her the treatment that in all likelihood would have saved her life. Not wanting to be an informer has accounted for many deaths under analogous circumstances, most of which could have been prevented by the timely use of blood transfusions and powerful, modern antibiotics.

Some women look upon the newly developing entity as a vampire sucking at the lifeblood of their own chances for future fulfillment, and in a frenzied state of anguish will do anything to abort themselves. It happened to one of my own research technicians. She was originally from Brazil, and was a member of a highly cultured family. She had been reared in a convent, as a devout Catholic. When she found herself pregnant, her lover departed to another country. She kept her condition secret for four months before confiding in a member of my staff, who referred her at once to a competent obstetrician. At this late stage in the pregnancy, he offered to care for her and deliver the baby. He also sent her for counseling. Shortly thereafter, she was absent from work. I knew nothing about her condition, but became concerned, because she was living alone. My secretary called her and found out she was ill, with a high fever. I sent someone to see her, and the story finally came out. Not being able to accept the obstetrician's advice, and anxious to rid herself of this pregnancy, she had injected herself with salt water through her abdominal wall, with a hypodermic needle more than four inches long. Luckily the water she introduced went into her womb, but hospitalization was required. After prolonged treatment with antibiotics and transfusions, her life was saved and the fetus aborted. But I was staggered at the emotional disturbance that would cause a person to take a long needle and, with no anesthesia, insert it blindly and deeply through her own abdominal wall.

Before the abortion laws were changed, when a woman was lucky enough to find a reputable doctor who would perform an abortion in spite of its illegality, the unfortunate victim might turn out to be the doctor. I was called on to testify against one of these, a brave man—and he *was* brave, his primary concern being that a woman determined to abort not be butchered by an amateur—early in 1952. As medical examiner, I had to be state's witness against a man highly respected for his kindliness and code of ethics. Dr. X had conscientiously and legally ministered to the needs of his patients for twenty-five years before the Westchester County grand jury indicted him on criminal charges of performing an illegal abortion and contributing to the delinquency of a minor.

The string of events terminating in Dr. X's downfall began when Phyllis Baylor, a seventeen-year-old high school senior, came to him for help. She was no stranger to Dr. X. He had officiated at her birth, had doctored her through all the usual childhood diseases, and had comforted her in periods of emotional stress. On this visit, Phyllis feared she was pregnant. Unwed, a minor, and not in tune with her parents' strict religious code, she turned to him rather than her parents. Dr. X examined her, and when he determined she was really pregnant, he convinced her to tell her parents. To ease her predicament, he arranged to talk it over with them and Phyllis in his office. After a lengthy discussion with the three of them, he suggested that they permit the pregnancy to go to term and then give the child to a recognized social agency for adoption. But now that their daughter was involved, the Baylors' religious code disintegrated: they asked Dr. X to arrange for a secret abortion. He would not advise them where they might get it done and actually had no access to or knowledge of any abortionists. He continued his efforts to dissuade them, but they remained adamant. Finally, concerned that Phyllis might fall into the hands of some incompetent or disreputable individual, and also aware of the emotional trauma she would suffer if exposed to an unsavory experience, he decided to take her into the accredited hospital where he was a staff member and do it himself. Under anesthesia and the best sanitary conditions, he performed the procedure in the operating room of the hospital. All approved hospitals require that all tissue removed in any surgical procedure be submitted to the pathology laboratory for analysis. The tiny fragments of tissue scraped from Phyllis' uterus were readily identified by the pathologist as the products of a conception. A permanent slide of this material was placed in the files of the department. When this finding was reported at the monthly meeting of the hospital's tissue committee (an established routine to check on all surgical procedures and prevent needless operations), Dr. X was summoned to the next meeting of this group and asked to explain his actions. Because of his previously unblemished record, he escaped with a severe reprimand but was warned that a repeat episode would lead to dismissal from the staff. He was instructed to wait, in the future, for the results of the laboratory test for pregnancy before proceeding with a curettage (an intrauterine scraping).

The matter might have ended there if Phyllis had not confided in her closest friend and told the entire story. The friend was dating a rookie cop, and in an unguarded moment betrayed Phyllis by relating all the details to him. This newly trained police officer, eager and anxious to make a mark for himself as an alert guardian of the law, reported the case to his commanding officer, who then relayed the information to the county district attorney.

Other doctors, who are not as straightforward as Dr. X, have in the past circumvented the anti-abortion law and carried out the procedure in established hospitals by subterfuge. The motivations of a few were as pure as were Dr. X's, but the majority of these doctors have done it for financial gain or to help "important" people. The doctor would prepare the would-be patient with a carefully rehearsed story to be told by her to the emergency-room doctor. Upon arrival at the hospital the patient would say she had been bleeding severely off and on for several days, and that she now was feeling some cramplike pains in the lower part of her abdomen. This simulated the story of an impending or spontaneous miscarriage, and it worked unless repeated too often. Or the patient would feign a psychiatric history and raise the possibility of suicide unless the pregnancy was ended. Psychiatric consultants, participants in the plan, would confirm the need for abortion. All of this was outside the law, but the law often looked the other way.

The district attorney had no choice but to proceed with a full-fledged investigation into Dr. X's behavior. At this point, I was requested to review the slides of the tissue on file at the local hospital to check on their accuracy. I determined that the tissue removed from the uterus of Phyllis Baylor by Dr. X revealed the products of a conception. Dr. X was found guilty of having performed an illegal abortion and sentenced on a felony charge. But in consideration of his previously unmarred record, and because Phyllis' father testified that the doctor had refused to accept a fee for his services, the sentence of one year in jail was suspended. Because this was a conviction on a felony charge, the case automatically was referred to the New York State Physicians Professional Conduct Committee, which suspended Dr. X's license to practice medicine for one year.

Here was a rare physician totally immersed in his patient's welfare—not interested in just today's acute aches and pains but in his patient's past, present, and future. This is a fast-vanishing breed of doctor, in spite of belated attempts at revival. To safeguard his patient and her chances for later fulfillment, Dr. X risked his career, reputation, and livelihood. He had probably never done an illegal abortion before. By my standards, he was a good physician.

American doctors have violently disagreed with each other about abortion. At one extreme has been the National Federation of Catholic Physicians, unanimously opposed to any attempt to liberalize any of the rigid anti-abortion laws. At the other end of the spectrum has been the Medical Committee for Human Rights, which has urged repeal of all the anti-abortion laws in every state. The Physicians Forum, also a liberal group but a more moderate one, believes there may be profoundly damaging social and psychological consequences to the mother, her family, and the child she bears when a woman is forced to continue an unwanted pregnancy. Older physicians, surprisingly, have a more liberal attitude than younger ones and in general have a more progressive attitude than the general public. Paradoxically, women physicians are more cautious and conservative on this subject.

Many doctors have been influenced by the effect liberal abortion laws have had on the health aspects of the problem. The overwhelmingly favorable experience with New York's liberalized law, with a striking drop in infant and maternal mortality and a sharp reduction in the number of births out of wedlock, should strengthen the hands of forces in other parts of the country. But putting questions of health aside, the stubborn focus of the Catholic Church on the two-celled embryo as a full-fledged human life, which no human being has the right to destroy, remains the basic obstacle to making abortion legal.

I had thought it best to stay away from the endless and unrewarding polemics on any of these side issues, but certain vital and glaring inconsistencies of the Church in these matters of life and death cry out for attention. On the simplest level, there is a known killer stalking this country—it is the cigarette habit. If the Church is so concerned about the mortal sin of taking human lives, why doesn't it excommunicate the makers, advertisers, and sellers of cigarettes, and the smokers themselves? The fact that cigarettes kill slowly and not quickly like an abortion does not alter the basic proposition.

On a more pertinent level, how can any faith, ethical code, religious body, or system of morality reconcile its horror over the death of a brainless, nerveless, heartless, eyeless, and earless microscopic speck of protoplasm with having condoned daily killings in Vietnam? The kind of sensibility that can reconcile these two things is beyond my ken; I can only report a conversation I had with a Filipino doctor I worked with. She had been raised a Roman Catholic and practiced her religion devoutly. Typically, she was vehement in her opposition to the then imminent passage of the New York abortion law. "In the eyes of God it is a mortal sin to take a life," she said. I asked her how, then, she could support our government's bombing of North Vietnam, which I had heard her do in strongly partisan terms. "Oh," she said, "but the North Vietnamese are Communists."

The courts, in some of their recent deliberations on abortion legislation, have legally defined life as beginning when the fetus possesses the capability for viability outside the womb. As a practical approach in seeking some resolution of the immediate controversy, this is as adequate a social definition as any. It is the one I have pragmatically adopted.

In January 1973, in a landmark opinion, the Supreme Court ruled, 7–2, that it was the right of a woman and her doctor to decide whether or not she should have an abortion during the first three months of pregnancy. Although still begging the basic question of the absolute right of the woman to decide (what about *after* the third month?), this victory technically overthrows most state laws prohibiting or restricting abortion. But the controversy isn't over. It will remain, certainly, for the near future. The counterattack has already begun: the court's decision has prompted plans to enact an anti-abortion amendment to the Constitution.

The overriding issue to me is that each woman must have the inviolate right to a complete freedom of choice as to how and what she will do with her own body and her own life. The other issues are all peripheral, an intellectual or emotional trick designed to camouflage or rationalize the hypocrisy, deep-rooted prejudice, antiquated theological dogma, or opportunistic political motivation that is aimed at keeping women shackled through outmoded abortion codes.

3. DOUBLE INDEMNITY—A QUESTION OF SUICIDE

"then is it sin
To rush into the secret house of death,
Ere death dare come to us?"

Shakespeare, ANTONY AND CLEOPATRA

No one ever lacks a good reason for suicide.

Cesare Pavese, THE BUSINESS OF LIVING

Suicide is a sensitive topic, since it is so bound up with guilt—not only the victim's guilt but also the guilt of the victim's relatives and the victim's doctor. The survivors always feel that, had they only done something differently, the victim would not have wanted to die.

My own first experience with suicide and guilt came while I was still a resident at Kings County Hospital. I was standing at the entrance to the hospital's admitting section after finishing a twelve-hour tour of duty. Someone shouted at me, "Look out." But before I could move, a man hurtled down from the roof above, his body falling so close that I felt the rush of air as he passed me. There was one brief cry as the man fell onto the iron grating above a shaftway, and then there was silence.

I rushed to the spot, to find that the impact of the man's fall had driven the grating down into the shaft below, and there, utterly destroyed, was the now lifeless body.

As I wandered, numb, back into the hospital, I heard one of the nurses saying she had seen the man, only moments before, enter the elevator in the main corridor mumbling: "No one cares for me. I am helpless, and I am alone." And suddenly, with a disquieting feeling, I knew he was the grubby little man who had tugged at my shirt; "I need help," he had pleaded. I had been examining another patient, and with hardly a glance upward at him, I had told him to sit down in the waiting room, that I would be with him in a few minutes. Undoubtedly confused, and feeling rejected because he had not received my immediate attention, he had wandered off and had last been seen alive by the nurse who had overheard his anguished appeal.

I immediately blamed myself for not having attended to the man's needs, for having been so preoccupied that I ignored his anxiety and the signs of impending disaster in his face. I accused myself of this needless death and wondered: if I had done this, or said that, or noticed something—if, if, and more ifs —perhaps this tragedy might have been averted. For months thereafter, at odd moments, my failure and my doubts would disturbingly emerge into my consciousness.

On the other hand, there are a number of suicides in which no one, no physician, no close friend, no intimate family member, is in a position to alter the course of events. Some people who have lived a good part of their lives without any overt signs of emotional disturbance or psychopathy become caught up in a rush of reversals and calamities often brought on by social pressure, distorted values, and basic dishonesty. The exposure of embezzled funds, fraud, mounting debts, and the possibility of imprisonment leads some of them to the conclusion that their only means of escape is suicide. These individuals plan the final, life-ending act as deviously and as carefully as they have their previous nefarious escapades. The surreptitious and well thought out execution of the suicide plan precludes any possibility of premature detection.

On one morning in August 1952 the state police notified my office in Westchester of the death of a thirty-nine-year-old restaurant manager. He had been struck and killed by an onrushing train on the Harlem Division of the New York Central Railroad, now the Penn Central. Apparently the victim had been in the process of changing a flat tire on the right rear wheel of his jacked-up car. The car was backed up to the end of a short dead-end road that stopped just before the railroad tracks. After a few more of the details of the mishap were relayed to me over the phone, I, like the cynical insurance-fraud investigator Keyes in Cain's novel *Double Indemnity* and like Edward G. Robinson in the film adaptation, suddenly experienced an uneasy feeling: Certain things just didn't sit right in the case.

The train engineer, in a statement taken at the scene of the fatality, gave his version of it: ". . . and then as I came around the bend a man suddenly appeared on the tracks and seemed to fling himself directly in the path of the train. There was no time to apply the brakes." Now, these words could be interpreted two ways. The man could have been looking for a rock or a block of wood to place in front of one of the wheels to prevent slippage of the car in the jacked-up position, and then, not noticing the train or reacting too late, could have been accidentally struck. The engineer might have deliberately misrepresented the event to cover his own negligence. Or it could have been a calculated suicide. Both were realistic possibilities.

There were, however, several facts I considered exceptional in what otherwise might be dismissed as either a routine suicide or an accident. First, as I was making the preliminary observations prior to doing the autopsy, I noticed that the back of the dead man's right hand was smudged with dirt, while the palm was clean. In contrast, the palm of the left was dirty, and the back was clean. It was as if he had used one hand to smear the other. At this point, I interrupted my examination, called the state police, and requested them to impound both the tire on the jacked-up wheel and the spare tire in the luggage compartment of the car and to check them for any defects. The second strange thing was the fact that the spare tire was still in the luggage compartment—it hadn't been removed before the car was jacked up. This, according to my way of doing things, was contrary to usual procedure. Also bothersome was the position of the car. Ordinarily, one would have driven a car with a flat tire head on directly into the dead-end road and changed the tire there, with the front end of the car facing the tracks. This man had carried out the more difficult maneuver of either backing into the dead-end road or turning around and then backing up to the railroad tracks at the end of the road.

Almost two hours later, the police reported back that both tires were perfect, free of any defects or leaks, and showed normal air pressure. To make doubly sure, they had inflated the tires under higher pressure and still there was no evidence of any escaping air. This enforced my original uneasiness. Now I dispatched Bill Roth, a veteran department investigator, to dig up as much background information as he could on the deceased. It began to take on the looks of a staged event—as if the victim were trying to disguise the suicide and make his death look like an accident. But why?

Within the next forty-eight hours Bill Roth supplied us with enough material to piece the affair together. The deceased had been the manager of the Yonkers branch of a well-known restaurant chain. The day before his death, a special audit of the restaurant's financial records had been completed and revealed a considerable shortage of funds. In addition, a local bank was demanding payment for a long overdue loan. Bill Roth discovered that the man had been spending considerable time at the racetrack, had incurred numerous gambling debts, and had been estranged from his wife for several months. Several weeks prior to his demise, he had insured himself, naming his wife and three children as the beneficiaries. The face value of this life insurance policy was fifty thousand dollars to be paid in the case of natural death, one hundred thousand dollars in case of accidental death. However, the policy also contained a special exclusion clause, which said that if the death was due to suicide all payment was automatically canceled—unless the policy had been in force for two years. This story was the usual sordid and sad one of a man with a wife and children, gambling debts, unpaid loans, embezzled funds, mounting personal pressures, and finally, as he saw it, no way out of shame, exposure, and imprisonment—and so suicide became the solution. Before terminating his life, he had had some remorse and made an effort to redeem himself by providing some financial security for his family. Even his last, heroic effort was fraudulent.

If this staged suicide had not been exposed, the family would have received the one hundred thousand dollars. The testimony of the train engineer, the absence of any defects in the tire, the seemingly contrived hand smudges, and the background of the personal and financial difficulties convinced me that this was a case of suicide. I certified it as such on the death certificate. The insurance company refused any benefit payments to the family on the basis of the suicide clause. Ultimately, the wife sued the insurance company, and the case ended up in court. The family contested my verdict. I was subpoenaed as a witness, and I testified as to my reasons for reaching a verdict of suicide. The jury upheld my official opinion and returned a decision in favor of the insurance company.

My friends have often asked me whether I feel guilty about playing a decisive part in depriving a widow and children of sorely needed financial aid that wealthy insurance companies could surely afford to pay. Like most people, my instincts are naturally on the side of the underdog. However, failure to come to terms with an issue such as this can lead to lack of objectivity and can tarnish the reputation of the medical examiners' office. The widow's problems cannot be solved by compromising with the truth. The only lasting solution lies in correcting the inequities in our social structure that allow for these situations. Sometimes the facts uncovered during an autopsy can help families; sometimes they cannot. Sometimes they help the insurance companies; sometimes they don't. In these instances, one's subjective feelings cannot be permitted to impede the search for the truth.

But the foregoing case is far from typical and is decidedly not representative of my over-all exposure to suicide. It is now my belief, after thirty years' experience with suicide, that there is considerable evidence to indicate that many doctors tend to underrate and deny the risk of suicide in their patients. I had not voiced this opinion until I read the report of the conference on iatrogenic (doctor-induced) diseases of the Medical Association of New Zealand. A well-known physician asked the question I had been asking myself: Why do so many suicidal patients, who are under medical care, commit suicidal acts? Isn't the doctor to blame for the dismal record? Isn't it possible that the psychology of the interpersonal relationship between a patient and his doctor could push the patient over the edge to self-destructive acts, if the patient feels decidedly unwanted by anyone? Professor W. Ironside, an authority in this area of study, spoke bluntly on the subject: "The doctor, having been antagonized by the patient, feels rejected himself and reacts with a depression which tends to project back onto the patient together with the suicidal impulse."

Twenty years ago, I had documented the salient characteristics of all reported suicides in Westchester County, and my findings had pointed to this conclusion: a doctor may be responsible for his patient's suicide. After reviewing the reports of the most recent international conferences on this subject, I see no reason to alter any of my original observations. More than half of the self-inflicted deaths among known psychiatric cases happened while the patients were either under the care of competent private psychiatrists or while they were in excellent mental hospitals. Some of the suicides took place shortly after the initial visit to a psychiatrist. Some killed themselves within a few days after being discharged from their doctors' care or from mental hospitals with a diagnosis of "improved—non-suicidal."

An absolutely typical case of this kind was that of an institutionalized twenty-four-year-old woman who had progressed so well from a deep depression that she was granted a weekend visit to her family. Thirty minutes after her departure from the hospital, we received a police call that she had been found dead after she had jumped from a nearby building. Her psychiatrist, when contacted for background information, was completely astonished and terribly upset. He had been sure that she was on her way toward recovery.

It is generally assumed that the frequency of suicides would be higher if it were not for the medical care received by potential suicide victims. It is difficult to estimate how many suicides have been prevented because of psychiatric care; accurate statistics for this are not available. Who knows how to define a suicide attempt? Something that may be thought an accident could have been intentional on the part of the victim; an incident thought to be a suicide attempt might be merely an accident. And how can anyone ever be sure that he has indeed prevented a suicide, and that in a week, or a year, or two years, the patient will not try again, with success?

The truth is that, in spite of recent progress in the care of the mentally ill, the suicide rate continues its inexorable rise. And we are still unable to recognize an impending individual suicide. Suicide on the personal level is unpredictable. We can describe the various methods people have used to commit suicide, but we don't always know why they did it; sometimes we can prevent a suicide, but we don't know whether or not we have succeeded in the long run.

About the only thing we do know for sure about suicide is that a certain number of people will commit suicide each year in a constant proportion according to social, economic, and geographic divisions. I cannot help feeling, as a result of being able to prognosticate so accurately the number of over-all suicides, that in the larger cosmos there is a highly specialized computer, meticulously and exquisitely programmed with all the hopes, frustrations, quirks, and frailties of human behavior, that punches out the proper number of deaths each year on the basis of population growth.

Statistics can tell us, for example, how many "self-inflicted fatalities" there will be; that twice as many men as women will kill themselves; that notes written and left by the victims will be found in one out of every three cases; that in the spring there is an increase in the number of suicides each year, and that there is a smaller but nonetheless real increase in suicides prior to the Christmas season; that more men than women will use violent methods, such as shooting and hanging; and that suicide by overdose of sleeping pills will be the most often used method.

What they don't tell us, and what we can't know, is which of the people surrounding us day by day are going to make up next year's statistics: Who among us today is going to try to commit suicide tomorrow? Will he or she succeed? Could the attempt be prevented? The peculiar human psychology that goes into the making of a suicide is shrouded, hidden deep within the mind of the individual. There must be something specific to human life that triggers an act of self-destruction, because human beings are the only animals that will take their own lives.

The statistics for the number of suicides per population unit are so constant and unrelenting that if something happens to disturb the proportion, human nature will find a way to restore the statistics to their proper balance. The case of "Good Gas" proved this to me.

In Westchester County, asphyxiation due to cooking gas had always been the second most frequent method of suicide—after barbiturate overdose. Typical was one year when, out of one hundred suicides, no fewer than forty-two had been committed with gas. But, in 1952, I began noticing over a period of months that not one suicide had been committed in this manner. By March 1953, one hundred twenty suicides had been committed, not one of them with gas. I grew suspicious. What was up?

It turned out that for the past year and a half, the manufactured gas previously delivered to Westchester had been replaced by natural gas. Manufactured gas is full of carbon monoxide, which has an even greater affinity for the body's hemoglobin than oxygen has. Natural gas is composed largely of methane and ethane, which do not replace oxygen in the blood. So it takes much more time, as well as much more gas, to kill oneself with natural gas. And in the time natural gas takes, most would-be suicides either change their minds or are discovered. This is what had happened in Westchester, and the statistics showed a corresponding drop in total suicides for that period.

But the decline was only temporary; by the end of the year, the expected number of suicides showed up in the statistics. Those who had failed because of the new, natural gas had tried again, but with a method more likely to insure success.

The unanswerable questions about suicide are heartbreaking, and the effort to somehow understand and live with the horror of it often drove the victims' relatives to me. In the course of my duties as medical examiner, I met and talked with husbands, wives, sons, daughters, fathers, mothers, lovers, and close friends of suicides, and in all of them similar gnawing questions persisted. The immediate aftermath of suicide—suffering, guilt, and shame—brought them to me, because, I suppose, I was the one who had rendered the final judgment, who had officially pronounced the loved one's death a suicide.

Especially in the case of parents, there is nothing so devastating and that imparts such an overwhelming sense of failure as a child's fatal act of self-destruction. Some parents would come to alleviate guilt, some to seek solace, some to challenge the correctness of my verdict, and others just to talk.

After our initial routine investigation into the suicide of a seventeen-year-old boy who had killed himself by hanging, I was paid a visit by his overwrought parents. From the family physician and the boy's older sister, we had learned that he had been afflicted with a minor disorder of the pituitary gland, a condition that had made him ungainly and large for his age. He had had little facility for athletics. He had had no close friends among his peers. He had been quiet and shy and had immersed himself with great intensity into boy-scout activities.

The father was middle-aged, partially bald, with precise features, piercing small eyes, and thin lips. He entered briskly, thrust out his hand, introduced himself, and in a voice big for his size, briefly stated the purpose of his visit. Meanwhile his wife, almost unnoticed, had unobtrusively followed him in. She was taller and had a kind face, but was otherwise nondescript. I remember it was late afternoon, because the low, setting autumn sun was streaming across my many-windowed room, and the feel of approaching winter further dampened my mood during what proved to be a very disconcerting session.

Without any further ceremony, he sat down and embarked upon a description of his late son. "He was a fine and obedient boy," he said. "He was well adjusted, did well in school, had no bad friends, never caused trouble. He didn't stay out late. He was not only a devoted boy scout, he scaled the heights by becoming an Eagle Scout. And yes, of course, he got along splendidly with his two older sisters."

And so he droned, on and on. During this exposition, the wife stared directly ahead, sometimes nodding in agreement and once or twice weeping silently. The father now began methodically to present his own virtues. "I have always been a concerned parent," he said. "I am always watching over my children." After a lengthy discourse designed to convince me of his excellence as a father, he related what he unquestionably considered to be the ultimate proof. "From the day my children were born, and to this very day, without fail, every night I have gone into their bedrooms with a flashlight and have conducted a careful bedcheck to be sure everything is safe and in order."

Previous exposure under similar circumstances to equally revealing and insensitive remarks had conditioned me to contain myself and not display any outward signs of dismay, so I did not react visibly to this. He then went on to describe the final hours in his son's life. The boy had had dinner at home, and then, in the company of his parents, he had gone into the living room to watch television. After about an hour of silence, he had bidden them goodnight and retired into his room.

The father claimed not to have observed, during these last

hours, anything suggestive of emotional disturbance or unhappiness in the boy. I silently observed that the father had been unaware of or had deliberately neglected to mention a fact I had learned from his sister: on the very same evening of the son's suicide, most of the girls and boys in the neighborhood were at a party in a house directly across the street. I never discovered whether the son had not been invited to this affair, or whether of his own volition he had chosen not to go. Is it conceivable that this father could have been completely oblivious to his son's loneliness and feeling of isolation on that evening? And then, as I had anticipated, he revealed the real motive for his visit. With a complete change in tone and now as if he were a lawyer summing up his case in court, he concluded that it must be obvious to me that the boy had been well adjusted and well behaved, and that he himself had been a proper and devoted parent. It should therefore be quite evident that my verdict of suicide by hanging in his son's death must be incorrect. He stated that he could not and would not accept as final my hasty judgment of his son's demise. He was convinced the death was accidental. "After all," he said, "my boy was a scout, and must have accidentally gotten strangled while practicing some new knots."

At this point I decided that the most constructive response was to refute this challenge and confront him with the facts. So, with great care and detail, I explained that the type of knot, the condition of the rope, the tight noose around the neck, the location and character of the rope pressure bruises (high in the neck beneath the ears), the position in which the body was found, and the manner in which the end of the rope was tied and hanging, could not conceivably have been accidental. However, I did concede that at times accidental stranglings do occur and have been mistaken for suicide. With reluctance, I explained that in my experience, as well as that of other medical

examiners, accidental stranglings sometimes involved a teen-
ager or a somewhat older person who had died from a mishap
after tying a rope around the neck to derive masochistic en-
joyment from the self-infliction of restraint and pain. These
were usually acts of sex perversion, and such subjects were
often found nude or clothed in women's attire with porno-
graphic or erotically posed nude females displayed in full view.
I decided to spare him one additional fact, that in these cases
there often is evidence of recent masturbation. The father,
totally unable to accept my unpalatable alternative explanation
for his son's death, now without hesitation accepted my original
verdict. He grabbed his wife by the arm and made a hasty exit.
This characterization of the father, his clichés, and his callous
lack of insight may appear crudely drawn, but, in so many of
my experiences, caricature and reality often blend so completely
as to be indistinguishable. Dramatic events are painted in broad
strokes.

Indeed accidental stranglings are rare, and aside from these
few examples of sex perversion, they usually occur in infants
who become inadvertently trapped in the rungs of a crib, or in
children whose necks have become entangled in window blinds
or in the ropes of a swing. Homicidal hangings are even more
unique, except, of course, decades ago, when lynchings were
commonplace. The deliberate suspension of a body after murder to simulate suicide is easily exposed at autopsy because
of the failure of the corpse to contain the telltale bruises,
abrasions, and small blood spots on the eyelids, scalp, and
neck, typically produced by hanging during life.

Fortunately in the past, suicide among adolescents was in-
frequent, and juvenile suicide was even less common. During
my five-year term as medical examiner in Westchester County,
there were no suicides under the age of fifteen. In this period,
only one out of every fifty suicides was in an individual under

twenty-one years. With advancing age, the number of cases rose sharply to reach a peak in mid-life. This personal but official experience was similar to observations on the national scene. Not only in the United Staes, but in other Western countries, the self-taking of life in children under the age of ten was almost unknown. Between the ages of ten and fifteen there were about fifty to sixty suicides a year in the entire United States. In Westchester, almost all these fatal acts were in boys, but in the entire country, one out of every three were in girls. At all ages, suicide still is more frequent in men, especially over sixty, when it occurs four times more often in men than in women.

Most experts agree that serious mental illness such as schizophrenia or psychotic depression accounts for only a fraction of these juvenile suicides. However, "staged suicidal attempts" in the young, without the real goal of death, are not uncommon, especially in girls. Accurate statistics on how often this happens are not available. Too often, the unsuccessful attempts at suicide are erroneously dismissed as showy gestures not to be taken seriously. The notion that the truly suicidal person must address himself to death alone dies hard. In fact, there are many psychiatrists who believe that most people who commit suicidal acts, fatal or not, do not want either to die or to live; they want to do both at the same time, usually one more or much more than the other. Past miscalculations have led to the sobering conclusion that all attempts or threats, no matter how exhibitionistic or inconsequential these may seem, must be viewed with concern. A great many of those who have completed the lethal act on themselves had records of previous threats or attempts.

The experts ascribed the infrequency of suicide in the young to a positive will to live and enjoy life, to get the most out of existence, and to venture, "with bold unconcern," into the unknown future. Youth possesses a growing curiosity, which is generally nourished by a continuous supply of new interests and expectation. There is always something to look forward to.

Nevertheless almost every month, I am asked by some lawyer representing a family to investigate the unnatural or unexplained death of a son or daughter. (Some of these prove to be drug or heroin poisonings—perhaps accidental, perhaps suicidal, or perhaps even homicidal.) This year alone I was involved with parents in this type of case in Providence, Denver, and San Francisco. Because I am not now working routinely in this particular field of pathology, and to keep abreast of any new developments, I recently consulted with my friend Dr. Henry Siegal, who was deputy chief medical examiner of New York. He had just completed a study on the increase in heroin and other drug-abuse deaths among New York City youth. One particular Sunday, the day's allotment of drug-abuse fatalities reposing on stainless-steel slabs in the chief medical examiner's office on First Avenue comprised five young men between the ages of eighteen and twenty-one. Dr. Siegal informed me that he was now often getting thirteen-year-olds dead of drug abuse and that while in 1966 there were only 33 heroin deaths among the New York City young, by 1969 the figure had risen to 224, and there were already 170 for just the first eight months of 1970. The precise number is inconsequential—only that the figures reflect a continuing upward trend. How many of these were suicides and how many were accidental overdoses remains undetermined. How many of these were basically the expression of a subconscious desire to end one's own life?

After all, what lies ahead for the present and future generations of youth? Because of the ever-accelerating pace of life, they have been permitted the fulfillment of almost every sexual experience before reaching maturity; the relative affluence of the middle class has left nothing for the youngster who has tasted lobster at the age of three and crepe suzettes at six. Santa Claus can no longer furnish any new delights or surprises for the youngster who has everything. Curiosity is blunted almost as soon as it is aroused, by the rapid dissemination of news and events via satellite and television. No one need leave the confines of the easy chair to view men in space, big-league baseball games, and riots in India at their very moment of inception; and by merely turning the knob on the television set, all three can be observed almost simultaneously.

Narrow and specialized technological training in industry and science diminishes the pleasure, the sense of self-esteem, and the chance of relating to the finished totality of any product or service. Some call this alienation. The fruits of personal achievement in science are perverted to pollute streams, contaminate the air, deface the mountains and trees, squander our natural resources, and destroy life. The results of cultural creativity are corrupted into crass and lying advertisements, television commercials, vulgarized art to sell soap, cigarettes, washing machines, and vitamin pills. And there is the growing and ever darkening shadow of the uncertainty of man's future life on earth. Today, the most knowledgeable and respected scientists seriously question whether in a decade from now there will be sufficient pure oxygen available in the atmosphere to meet our daily needs for survival. Hovering over all this is the ever-pervasive and mind-blowing threat of total extermination: the proliferous stockpile of increasingly powerful nuclear bombs, which can already demolish the earth one hundred times over, grows daily. Columbia University's noted biochemist Professor Erwin Chargaff stated it clearly: "There is no question in my mind that we live in one of the truly bestial centuries in human history. There are plenty of signposts for the future historian, and what do they say? They say 'Auschwitz' and 'Dresden' and 'Hiroshima' and 'Vietnam' and 'Napalm.' For many years we have all been waking up to the daily body count on the radio; and if there were a way to kill people with the B Minor Mass, the Pentagon-Madison Avenue axis would have found it." If society puts so little value on human life, how can this but thwart any positive will to live? In addition to instant rice, instant coffee, instant soup, instant spot removers, instant muffins, we have instant satisfaction of curiosity, instant fulfillment of imagination, instant growth, instant change, instant success, instant mind expansion, instant revolution, instant war, and finally instant extermination. This plastic life mix is then trimmed with a cultural icing prepared from a recipe whose ingredients include the modern novel featuring the non-hero, the non-person, and the non-story; the modern theater presenting the absurd, the meaningless, and the non-verbal plays of Grotowski; a graphic art lacking in sentiment, full of pop, and accompanied by the non-music of Cage, utterly devoid of melody or tonality. It is logical that the Nobel Prize in Literature would be awarded to Samuel Beckett, whose predominant theme is "the futility of modern life." Is there any wonder that reality lacks meaning and nothing is real? So we witness increasing numbers of youth in their flight from substance into astrology, nirvana, Scientology, the worship of the guru, meditation, beat, hip, Zen, LSD, speed, grass, heroin, glue, hashish, and banana skins. Can such a potpourri ignite and fuel a sufficient life force? Or are we now harvesting a flourishing crop of youthful suicides and "cop-outs"? The name of the London musical show *Stop the World I Want to Get Off* becomes a real but sinister wish: After all, the taking of drugs by rich, white, suburban youth is symptomatic of a desire to escape from what they feel is a futile and meaningless world into unreality, and this is not very far short of a wish for death.

Dr. Siegal mentioned to me that half the cases of death due to drugs were black youths. It seems highly probable to me that these deaths were, at least subconsciously, suicides; the reality of the black ghetto, with its violence, dehumanization, degradation, drug addiction, maternal deprivation, and hopelessness is driving increasing numbers of black youth to suicide.

Suicide in the Negro population used to be relatively rare: in Westchester County, from 1945 to 1955, Negro suicides accounted for only one out of every one hundred, despite the fact that Negroes represented more than 5 per cent of the county's population. In recent years I had been aware of an increase, but I was startled to learn that in 1967 in New York City the rate had jumped spectacularly; the suicide rate was twice as high among Negro men between twenty and thirty-five as it was among white men in the same age group.

Over fifty years ago, Sigmund Freud considered suicide to be an inverted form of homicide. This was interpreted by many to mean that the desire to kill oneself was really an outgrowth of an unconscious desire to kill someone else. Violent rage developed from years of racism and degradation is manifested externally in such destructive episodes as ghetto burnings and riots, but can also be turned inward to destroy one's own life. Of course, without any consideration of cultural and ethnic differences and problems, generalizations about suicide are precarious.

In the past decade, along with the recent increase in the suicide rate among teen-agers, there has also been a gradual but distinct increase in the suicide rate in men over the age of sixty-five. Excerpts from some of the suicide notes give the reasons:

"I always knew that I would end my life as soon as I found that I was a burden on others."

"There is no point in going on. I am no longer working, I cannot produce anything, I am just existing."

"When I try to move, the pain I get in my heart is too much, so goodby."

"No charity for me, no sir."

"I'd sooner be ashes than ask for help."

Many men, having been taught that their sole purpose in life is to support and to care for a family, feel painfully unneeded after retirement. Their sons and daughters seldom help them cope with their real problems. The old are too often left to their memories in a society that relegates "senior citizens" to "leisure villages."

Self-destructive acts in the elderly are rarely seen in women, because the deeply ingrained Protestant work ethic fixes the responsibility for self and family firmly on the male and does not frown on a woman who does not work or who cannot care for herself. Women also are better endurers of pain, so they rarely kill themselves for reasons of incurable or chronically painful disease. This is in part why I have always seriously maintained that women are the stronger sex. To me, the claim that men are stronger is a myth—entirely unsupported by any facts.

The many former friends and relatives of suicide victims with whom I talked were most concerned about the question of predictability. This was succinctly expressed by a woman whose husband had just shot himself, when she asked, "Was I too self-absorbed with my own problems, and was I so unaware of his torment, and so blind as not to detect anything— any sign which might have made me sense the imminence of my husband's suicide?" What this woman and others have asked and continue to ask is the crucial question. Can doctors or psychiatrists recognize the potential suicide victim in time to interrupt the fatal completion of the act? And if they can do this, are they then able to defuse the ever-present time bomb hanging over the lives of these individuals?

A meeting with a Catholic priest over the wording on a cer-

tain death certificate helped me to answer these questions. In
my first week as medical examiner, I had certified the death
of a middle-aged Catholic man as "Suicide caused by self-
inflicted gunshot wound of the head." The same day, shortly
thereafter, a young Roman Catholic priest from a Yonkers
parish came to discuss the wording on this death certificate.
He discreetly explained that he had no desire for me to alter
my professional evaluation of this or any other case. He then
told me something I should have known but of which I confess
complete ignorance at that time. The Catholic Church regards
the taking of one's own life as a sin, and for this reason the
victim cannot be buried with the full blessings of the Church.
With this explanation, he politely suggested a solution to this
dilemma. He said if I would simply add to my statement already
on the certificate of death the following words: "while temporarily mentally disturbed," the Church would be satisfied. This
was the arrangement the Roman Catholic Church had had
with my predecessor, Dr. Squires, and also with many other
medical examiners and coroners throughout the country. With
this simple addition, it would now be possible for the deceased
to be buried with the full sacraments. I suddenly realized that
that was the way I felt about suicide too, and that it certainly
was no distortion or compromise with the truth to add, "while
temporarily mentally disturbed." No matter how long a troubled
individual may brood, plan, and contemplate over whether to
take his life, the ability to consummate self-destruction requires
at least a moment of complete irrationality. Therefore, if the
actual act of killing oneself is insane, how can any rational perception detect something so devious, spontaneous, and tortu-
ous? Human actions are so deeply influenced by the individual's
past that they appear irrational, and hence, usually unpredictable. How, then, can we predict the unpredictable, or succeed
with logic in an illogical situation? We cannot, in short, hope

to predict an individual's propensity toward suicide with any accuracy.

The precarious and fragile balance that exists between a disturbed person's life force and his drive toward self-negation may be upset by the well-intentioned but amateur meddler. Too often, the relatives or friends are unaware of the dynamics involved in the potential suicide. This lack of understanding leads them to believe that the sheer force of their own personalities and powers of persuasion can instill sufficient motivation and strength into the mentally sick. They really believe that by the positive transfer of will a person can be transformed from a vegetative to an actively functioning state and can thus break out of his feelings of inadequacy and despair.

A case in point was the cashier of a local bank who could not comprehend his wife's suicide. They had been married for two years, and there were no children. Several months prior to her death, she had become apathetic and could not function properly. The family physician advised hospitalization. She had been in the hospital about two weeks when the husband visited her, gave her a pep talk, and insisted that she come home to resume her wifely duties. He demanded she be discharged. Against the doctor's advice, she was discharged, and a few days later committed suicide.

Her husband came to see me in a state of profound grief and bewilderment. He could not understand why she took her own life. She had been, he said, such an excellent housekeeper and cook before her illness. After her discharge from the hospital, he had exhorted her, every morning before he went off to work, to get on with her daily chores, just as had been her wont. He indicated to me that he had insisted that she start doing her work again. "I don't understand how she could have done this to me, how she could have left me to be alone. I gave her such a good home." This attempt to stimulate positive ac-

tivity into his depressed wife had accentuated the disparity between her recent ineffectiveness and her former skillful ability
to satisfy his domestic and personal needs, thus bringing her
to a breaking point that may well have precipitated the final act.

More understandable, from the standpoint of predictability,
are the periods in history when social and economic upheavals
appreciably alter the suicide rate. The catastrophic depression
of the early 1930s brought forth a rash of suicides. Almost
daily, bodies plummeted down from the parapets and rooftops
of Wall Street empires. Of telltale significance was the fact that
these deaths were almost entirely limited to men aged thirty-
five to fifty-five. The old, the young, the black, the women
were untouched. The average working man was not moved to
suicide even though he had lost his job. The phenomenon was
confined to men relatively high in the social and economic
ladder who because of financial loss were reduced from three
limousines to one or from a large estate to a small apartment.
Joblessness, poverty, dispossession into the streets, or elemental
deprivation did not drive men to end their lives. It was the
loss of power, loss of social status, tormented vanity, and false
pride—all false idols—that induced the crack-up in these men
at the peak of their careers.

Louis Dublin, the renowned statistician for the Metropolitan
Life Insurance Company, authored a book on suicide entitled
To Be or Not to Be, in which he described the profile of suicide
during this period for the country as a whole. World War II
witnessed a decline in the domestic suicide rate—in the same
segment of men in which it had increased during the depression.
Again, the other groups were unaffected. This drop has been
attributed to the intense and collective involvement in a massive national effort which jolted these men out of self-pampering
attitudes and redirected their attention away from their inner,
personal worries. In both these periods, depression and war, the

suicides that were caused by serious mental disease remained entirely unaffected: these rates did not go up or down.

The influence of cultural change on national suicide rates is illustrated by post-World War II Japan, where there has been a considerable reduction in the number of suicides in the decades since the war. This reduction has coincided with the disillusionment of the younger generations toward the age-old question of "saving face," which in the past necessitated hara-kiri.

A look into other aspects of suicide patterns offers an opportunity for romantic speculation, but little to unravel the sphinx-like riddle. The tendency for more attempts at suicide to occur during the early spring season can play havoc with one's imagination. If one is so inclined, he might attribute the seasonal rise in suicides to the ides of March. Others could invoke the force of astrology: After all, this increase coincides with the sign of the fish, Pisces, in which two fish are seen swimming in opposite directions. This could be interpreted to mean a lack of purpose or confusion in one's life goals. People born under this sign are said to be easily addicted to drugs and alcohol. Aries, in the very next period—also in spring—is the sign of the ram. This is a fire sign. Could this possibly mean that individuals under this sign tend to be consumed in the flames of their own passions? Surely these metaphysical assumptions are just as valid as many psychoanalytic interpretations of suicide. My favorite explanation is rather simplistic and free of any profound psychoanalytic theories. It seems to me that severely depressed individuals, full of despair and waning hope, are unable to cope with the contrasting reality of new life and hope emerging from the ground and suffusing the air during the early spring season. The widening chasm between their hopeless life and new life emerging deepens the depression to a point that precipitates the suicide. This same pattern of increase in suicides in early spring has also been observed in Great Britain. Down under, in Australia, however, where the seasons are reversed and our autumn is their spring, the suicides rise in September and October and drop during March and April. For a brief period prior to the Christmas season, there is again a slight rise in the number of suicides in all Christian countries. The inability to cope with the surrounding gaiety and family reunions at this time of year seems to accentuate a tendency toward self-destruction.

Like so many others, I became intrigued with the study of suicide notes, hoping to gain from this a deeper understanding of the problem. These messages from the dead to the living are found in about one third of all suicides. Twice as many men as women leave them. This is understandable, as the contents often spell out the final arrangements to be made concerning unfinished business and financial affairs. It is certain that more notes are written and left than we are aware of. Members of a family, coming upon them first, often destroy or conceal them for many reasons—some in order to disguise the nature of death, and others because of the highly personal contents of the note. Because suicide is legally considered a criminal act, the notes are regarded as primary evidence, and, when I was a medical examiner, the originals were always sent to our office for permanent safekeeping. Upon request from the district attorney's office, or from relatives or authorized legal representatives, we supplied duplicates of these notes. These messages varied considerably. At one end of the scale were many short, unintelligible, and incoherent scrawls on scraps or bits of paper, and at the other end of the scale were the ones that were lengthy, literate, logical, and convincing. The messages contained expressions of love, hate, despair, and relief. Some were plaintive appeals and some were defiant. In one instance, there was a note addressed and left for the suicide victim's dog. Key sentences or phrases from some of these notes reveal the wide range of emotion: "Don't pity me—I pity you." "The fear was too much to bear." "Please forgive me, but this is best for everyone." "Perhaps now you will finally miss me." "I hate to do this to you, but there is no alternative for me." "Say goodby to the boys for me." "Farewell, you never knew it, but I have always loved you dearly." "You did this to me, I hate you, I hate you." "Play it cool baby." "Quick, quick, like a bunny." And finally the note to the dog: "Bow wow and goodby, Pepper."

The contents of one note has remained with me to this day. It was a poignantly set forth narrative describing with sensitive passion the main events in this seventy-four-year-old man's life. He had been a successful book-publishing executive. In this document, which could almost have been published as a short story, he related his fifty years of idyllic relationship with his wife. She had died just two months previously. His professional and business career had left him content, fulfilled, and in financial security. He discussed all of this. He concluded that, now that his wife was dead, he was retired from his work, had no children, and was in frail health, each day became a dragging and dull reduplication of the previous one. He was almost reduced to elemental biological existence stripped of all human overtones—except for memories, and these, too, were rapidly becoming obscure, distant, and befuddled. So, he explained with incontrovertible logic, it was time to call a halt to his life. This narrative convinced me of the rationality of his final decisive act.

Only recently, at an international conference on the subject of suicide prevention, during the summer of 1971, an eminent physician defended the right of an individual to end his own life. He condemned the self-righteousness, and the morality, that sometimes frustrate these attempts. After all, he said, if we concede that the individual has the right to personal self-determination, and the right to live his life in his own way, so we must also concede that his right to die at a time of his own choosing and in his own manner must also be inviolate. He concluded by challenging anyone to deny the supremacy of Socrates' intellect, a man who, when he recognized the futile meaninglessness of his own continued existence, took hemlock.

On the evidence of suicide notes, taken at face value and without any speculative probes into their inner or deeper symbolic meanings, we must conclude that suicide is a many-headed thing. It is a synthesis of multiple contradictions composed of such opposites as love and hate, defiance and acceptance, courage and cowardice, logic and illogic, anguish and relief, arrogance and humility, egocentricity and selflessness, scorn and pity. Emotionally it is one and all of these things. Yet, on the most elemental biological level, where the only meaning of life is life itself—the struggle for survival and its perpetuation—this taking of one's own life must be regarded as a complete negation, utterly insane and without meaning. The more biological and the less human our lives are, the more we merely toil only for the next day's survival. But the more human our lives are, the more vulnerable and sensitive we become to the surrounding pressures. Suicide is, indeed, a peculiarly human affair.

III

MADISON AVENUE MURDERS

1. THE CIGARETTE-SMOKING CONTROVERSY

The wretcheder one is, the more one smokes: the more one smokes
the wretcheder one gets—a vicious cycle.

George L. P. B. Du Maurier, PETER IBBETSON

I should say at the start that I am vehemently anti-cigarette.
I've done research on lung cancer and was a member of the
first National Study Group on Smoking and Health. I am not
going to talk about the physical evidence linking smoking to
lung cancer; enough has been said about it, and there are few
people who haven't read either the Surgeon General's report
or a cigarette pack, both of which say: "Warning: The Surgeon
General Has Determined That Cigarette Smoking Is Dangerous
to Your Health."

Little has been said, though, about the machinating that prevented this evidence from reaching the public until it became
embarrassing for the machinators not to release it. It is probably this political angle, which allowed a vested interest to inter-
fere with the public's right to know, even more than my desire
to save lives, that has made me want to see the tobacco industry tried for murder.

This fanciful wish was almost realized at the very beginning of the battle against smoking, in 1958, when the widow of a man who had died of lung cancer sued the tobacco company that made the brand of cigarettes he had smoked. She asked me to be one of five medical witnesses, and I agreed. I felt rather strange about it; a federal courthouse in New Orleans seemed the least likely place for me to be debating the scientific case against cigarettes. For me, as for most scientists, the proper place for such a discussion has always been the clinic, the laboratory, or the university conference room.

This case had been conceived and initiated by one of the nation's most distinguished chest surgeons, Dr. Alton Ochsner, of New Orleans. He had not only been president of the American College of Surgeons, but was one of the pioneers in suggesting a close connection between smoking and cancer. The deceased had been a patient of Dr. Ochsner's, and he convinced the widow to start the legal proceedings. He also secured the attorney and selected the medical witnesses.

Years ago, Dr. Ochsner created a stir in medical circles when he said: "During my medical-student days, I saw only one lung-cancer case in four years. Today I operate on from two to four such cases every week. Now when I see a patient whose symptoms suggest lung cancer and who has been a heavy cigarette smoker, I make a tentative diagnosis of epidermoid lung cancer—or what has come to be known as smoker's cancer. Thus far, I have been right in 95 per cent of these diagnoses." Most doctors refused to take him seriously.

The legal basis for the action was brought under the implied-warrant-of-safety concept inherent in common law. The federal court in Louisiana was a favorable jurisdiction for this important test case, because Louisiana law still embodies the traditions of the old Napoleonic code, dating from its French colonial period. This code permits a broad interpretation of common-law practices; in this case, it would allow broad inter-

pretation of the implied guarantee of safety for any product sold
for human use in a public place.

The chief attorney for the plaintiff, William Brumfield, was
a short, stocky, red-bearded, and sharp-witted man from Baton
Rouge. Together with Dr. Ochsner, he met with the panel of
medical experts in New York to outline the strategy for the
case. Among those present were Dr. Ernest Wynder, who is
both an experimentalist and epidemiologist specializing in lung
cancer and the head of a section in the famous Sloan-Kettering
cancer institute; Dr. Mort Levin, from Roswell Park State Cancer Hospital and the state Department of Health; and Dr.
Dean Davies, who had been the executive secretary of the
National Study Group on Smoking and Health.

After listening to Dr. Ochsner outline his reasons for bringing this case to trial, we all agreed to testify. I can't speak for
the others, but I refused to accept a fee (although I agreed
to be recompensed for travel and hotel expenses). Most of us
present that day did not believe this was the best way to settle
a scientific problem, but, bowing to the inevitable fact that the
case was going to trial, we thought we should make the best
possible presentation of all the facts in court. The nation would
be following this trial closely. We were convinced that the entire
tobacco industry would spare nothing in its defense. They could
not risk losing one such case.

Mr. Brumfield explained to us that if we could show that
the cigarette manufacturer had breached an implied warranty
of fitness for human consumption, the company would be held
responsible for the death or disease of the cigarette consumer.
On the surface, it seemed simple to prove to the jury that cigarettes actually caused cancer and were not safe for human consumption. But Mr. Brumfield then enumerated the complexities
involved in trying to establish this in court. The most difficult
problem to overcome was the fact that most people change their

cigarette brands a number of times during their smoking career. This raises the issue of which brand is responsible for the cancer, and whether it is possible to absolutely incriminate any one brand in particular.

Furthermore, in civil litigation, the law makes unreasonable demands upon the scientist or doctor by asking that inevitable question, "Can you testify with reasonable medical certainty that a disease was caused by a specific given factor and was not caused by something else?" There are rarely absolute answers to this question, and the lack of them often leads to the art of gamesmanship in court. Unfortunately, there are those physicians who will commit themselves to absolute statements that are not scientifically justified, either because of ignorance of all the facts or because of their desire to assist in a favorable verdict. In some instances, it is because of the remuneration.

My assignment was to present testimony, derived from studies on human autopsies, that would show the connection between the cancer-producing chemicals known to be present in cigarette smoke and the abnormal alterations in the lining of the bronchial tubes. I was to trace the progress of the cancer from the earliest cellular changes to the fully developed growth. I was also supposed to demonstrate how some of these chemicals caused similar kinds of cancer when introduced experimentally into animals.

Several more strategy sessions were held in New York. At one of these, Melvin Belli, the noted negligence attorney from the West Coast, joined the plaintiff's legal team. This troubled me personally, because Mr. Belli had a national reputation for obtaining huge financial verdicts for his clients in malpractice suits against doctors.

Two days before the date set for the trial, we all assembled in New Orleans. My wife, who had never been to New Orleans, came with me at my own expense. As it turned out, it was a good thing she did. Her presence was, for me, the saving grace of the entire venture.

Selection of the jury had begun; the nation's press representatives were there in full force; and the cigarette industry had engaged a remarkably large array of expensive legal talent. The press was reporting every detail. On the second day, while we were sitting at lunch, someone brought the afternoon edition of a New Orleans newspaper, just off the press, over to our table. There, in two-inch letters across the entire front page, was the headline: FEDERAL JUDGE DECLARES MISTRIAL IN SMOKING CASE—JURY TAMPERING CHARGED. We couldn't believe it. The trial was over before it had ever started. The months of intense preparation had all been for nothing. No new date for the trial was set; it was postponed indefinitely. Bringing a case to trial is a very complicated affair, and this case never did come to trial again.

We learned that a private investigator hired by Messrs. Brumfield and Belli had telephoned relatives, neighbors, and friends of prospective jurors to find out the smoking habits of the jury panel. One of the jurors reported this to the judge, who called a hearing with counsel for both sides and declared a mistrial. This sudden and unexpected termination of the trial bothered me. It was too easy, too pat. I have always wondered if somewhere there had been a deliberate fix. A victory in this trial, if sustained in the higher courts, could have set a precedent that had the potential of financially ruining the cigarette industry. There was too much involved for me to naïvely accept such a stupid ending to the case.

Within the year, there were a flurry of similar cases pending in the courts in various parts of the country. In three of them, one from Pittsburgh, one from California, and one from Florida, I was called by the attorneys to participate, but only one of these—the Florida case—actually materialized. The attorneys for both sides and the court reporters traveled from Florida to my office in New York and took sworn testimony from me, to spare me the trouble of going down. The examination, under oath, consisted of direct examination by Lawrence Hastings, the plaintiff's lawyer; a cross-examination by defense counsel, of which there were two; and redirect affirmation, again by Mr. Hastings. It took three hours. I was questioned exhaustively on all the evidence linking smoking to cancer of the lungs. In a crucial point, the defense counsel tried to show that whatever alleged evidence was known was of recent vintage and not generally available or acceptable more than five years before. I disagreed with this, and felt certain I had offered enough facts to prove that the case against cigarettes had been established long before that and that there had been a sufficient lapse of time for the cigarette manufacturers to do something about it.

In August of that year, 1960, I received a letter from Mr. Hastings thanking me for my services in which he said, "I am sure that some word has probably reached you with regard to the results of our trial. We achieved, through your great and humane efforts, what I believe and hope will be a far-reaching 'victory.' Unfortunately, however, as you will see by the enclosed clippings, we did not receive any monetary award. The jury found his smoking caused his lung cancer, but they felt the tobacco company did not have sufficient knowledge to prevent the injuries prior to February 1, 1956—the date the plaintiff's biopsy showed cancer."

Ironically, the subsequent government regulation requiring cigarette packages to carry a warning label that cigarettes are hazardous to health did little to curb smoking but took the manufacturers off the hook and protected them from any further litigation on the issue of implied warranty. In other words, it was now clear that people smoked at their own risk.

But what about the risk to the non-smoker—what about his

civil rights? In 1972 the Surgeon General, in his annual report, pointed up the harm to non-smokers from the smoke of nearby smokers. Among the allergies suffered were watery eyes, nasal blockage, and severe headaches. He mentioned that some of the allergies could be quite extreme. The Non-Smokers Liberation movement received a boost from this report and has become more active and articulate in its demands.

Approximately one million lung-cancer deaths have been reported in this country alone since the day I saw a case of lung cancer for the first time—over thirty years ago, at the Baltimore City Hospital. Dr. Frank Geraghty, our clinical instructor, was in the midst of teaching a small group of medical students the technique of chest examination. An intern interrupted our class to announce an upcoming autopsy of a suspected lung-cancer case. Because lung cancer was almost an oddity in those days, Dr. Geraghty did not want us to miss this opportunity, so he suspended the class. By the time we arrived in the dissecting room, there was standing room only—a real testimony to the uncommonness of this disease. At that time, in the whole country, there were fewer than three thousand such cases observed annually, which meant there were only five cases for that year in the entire city of Baltimore. Malignant tumors of the lung rose to eighteen thousand by 1950 and then to over fifty thousand annually in 1965. This rate of increase is unparalleled by any other form of cancer. Public-health experts now call this an epidemic of major proportion, with the end not yet in sight.

The consumption of cigarettes in the United States did not become a major threat to man's health until the early 1920s. Since World War I, sales have expanded fivefold. About four billion cigarettes were manufactured in 1900, but currently five hundred billion are produced annually.

In a very real sense, the history of the controversy over cigarette smoking is an incisive portrayal of our society's prevailing morality. It is replete with political intrigue, financial manipulation, distorted news reports, communications-media censorship, heated and often infamous scientific debate, civil litigation, fraudulent publications, human indifference, and downright intellectual dishonesty. Without subscribing to the devil theory of history, I nevertheless feel that the smoking saga reflects the conflict between those motivated by materialism and self-seeking and those trying to get on with the job of improving the quality of human life.

I do not mean to imply that, in the absence of self-interest, the nation's smoking habits would be easily altered. The deeply ingrained cultural patterns and the chronicity of the habit indeed require a prolonged, determined, and massive approach. And up till now it has not been possible to mount the kind of mammoth campaign needed to pass on the benefits of research that correlates lung cancer and smoking. Also, it must be noted that cigarette smoking is not the only cause of lung cancer. Today we must contend as well with air pollution and with occupational exposure to irritants such as asbestos and uranium.

During the 1940s, as pathologist for the Chest Disease Division at Bellevue Hospital, I first became aware, as did many others at that time, of a striking statistical association between cigarette smoking and lung cancer. This form of cancer was rarely discovered at the autopsy table in non-smokers. Because of this, Dr. Herbert Maier, a leading pulmonary surgeon at the hospital, hesitated before ever making a definite diagnosis of this malignancy in anyone who had never smoked cigarettes. In face of this mounting evidence, we began to teach our findings to medical students, but few took them seriously. Jar upon jar filled with lung-cancer specimens began to line the shelves in my laboratory.

This extensive exposure led me to make some personal investigations into the problem. It was probably this study of mine

—which I am still conducting—that prompted an invitation from a national body of scientists to join them in a review and report on all aspects of the relation between smoking and cancer. The National Study Group on Smoking and Health was formed in 1955, at the instigation of Dr. Leroy E. Burney, then Assistant Surgeon General of the United States. It was sponsored by the National Cancer Institute, the National Heart Institute, the American Cancer Society, and the American Heart Association, and comprised seven men, representing the fields of chemistry, statistics, cancer research, heart-disease research, lung-disease research, pathology, and toxicology.

After two years of careful, critical, and firsthand scrutiny of at least sixteen independent research projects carried on in five different countries (with the primary investigators appearing before us to present their original findings and to debate with their critics), we formulated some definitive conclusions and suggested areas of still-needed research. Because the study group realized the far-reaching implications of our conclusions on both the country's habits and the nation's economy, we refused to release any information until the details of the deliberations were reviewed and evaluated by the governing scientific boards of the four sponsoring organizations. Only after their unanimous concurrence with our findings and the wording of our report was the study to be officially released—and then it would be released not to the press but as a co-operative report in *Science,* the official journal of the American Association for the Advancement of Science.

But before this correct and orderly procedure could be completed, someone leaked the contents of the study group's appraisal to the Atlanta *Constitution* and then to the wire services. This occurred while the board of directors of the American Cancer Society was meeting in Atlanta to assess the study group's conclusions and to pass final judgment.

A telegram from Dr. Heller, director of the National Cancer Institute, informed me of this breach and released the members of the group from our pledge to maintain the confidentiality of our findings. As soon as I finished reading the telegram, I received a call from Harold Schmeck, science reporter for the New York *Times*. He said he had been authorized by the American Cancer Society to contact me and asked if I could meet with him to discuss the report, fragments of which had already come over the wire services and been printed in the Atlanta paper. After a consultation with Dean Davies, the permanent executive officer of the study group, a meeting was arranged, and I agreed to co-operate with Mr. Schmeck—on condition that the New York *Times* publish the entire text of the report to minimize the possibility of misinterpretation or distortion of its contents.

That afternoon, the American Cancer Society delivered the full text to the *Times* office, where I was being interviewed. The next morning, Saturday, March 23, 1957, the report, along with a short biographical résumé of the study group's members, was featured on the front page of the paper. The report stated, ". . . the sum total of scientific evidence establishes beyond reasonable doubt that cigarette smoking is a causative factor in the rapidly increasing incidence of human epidermoid cancer of the lung."

Following the publication of our findings in the New York *Times*, I was deluged with calls from local newspapers, radio stations, and the public in general (I was the only one of the study group who lived in New York). It seemed that, with this disclosure, a battle was now being joined in earnest. This was the first national pronouncement by a semiofficial body condemning cigarettes as hazardous to health. Backing these conclusions was the prestige of the foremost national scientific organizations in the country. Reacting were the tobacco interests and their dependents.

But before delineating the line-up of the opponents, some thoughts on the leakage of the findings seem relevant to an understanding of the kind of struggle that was to emerge in this anti-cancer crusade. (I hasten to add that these are entirely personal speculations derived to some extent from certain rumors and stories widely circulated at that time.)

The study group itself had been pledged to secrecy. There was no reason to believe that any member had broken his pledge. The boards of the sponsoring organizations, conservative, responsible, and keenly aware of the implications, were committed to a joint report to appear at a later date. Logic seemed to dictate that the cigarette industry as a whole had no desire for any widespread publicity to be given to our report, because this might at least temporarily cut back on the consumption of their product. Who, then, was responsible for this precipitous and unexplained disclosure?

My feeling was that it was the work of a small group of stockholders in the cigarette industry who conspired to make a quick financial gain by playing both ends against the middle. They correctly anticipated that the release of any information adverse to cigarettes would produce a sharp drop in the price of cigarette-company shares on the stock market. Forewarned, they sold a large block of shares prior to the prearranged publication of the report on Friday. At the close of the stock market that Friday, the shares of all the major cigarette manufacturers did actually decline several points, and by Monday, after the full impact of the national publicity, their prices dropped even lower. At this point, these original shareholders then repurchased an equivalent or perhaps even a larger block of shares. They now owned at least as much stock as before, with a tidy profit gained from the difference between the sale and repurchase price. A neat trick, and not uncommonly practiced over the years—especially by unscrupulous and astute manipulators of the market. This kind of transaction is now against the law, but it must be proved to have been planned in advance.

The major forces impeding the implementation of an anti-cigarette campaign have been and continue to be primarily those with a financial interest—those dependent upon an uninterrupted increase in the sale of cigarettes. They include the six hundred thousand farm families who (in 1963) received $1,154,000,000 for their cigarette tobacco—only about two thousand dollars apiece; the cigarette manufacturers, who in a single year collected $1,408,000,000; the shippers, distributors, and vendors, who annually receive $7,288,000,000; the various governmental divisions that collect taxes on tobacco (the federal government collects approximately $2,047,000,000 a year, New York State $1,201,000,000, New York City $72,000,000); and the communications media, which in 1967 alone took in $311,900,000 in cigarette revenues (with television getting the lion's share, $226,900,000). With these powerful interests lobbying for cigarettes and cigarette advertisements the anti-smoking campaign had a hard time getting started.

Defects in the nation's medical-school curriculums, the ignorance and apathy of too many doctors, and the deliberate foot-dragging of some of the major sections of organized medicine also served the cause of "anti-health." The governmental officials of the major tobacco states, in the South, and their representatives in Congress, were and still are important reserves in this battle. To further complicate the whole affair was the double-edged role of the federal government at this time, which simultaneously financed (via the National Institutes of Health) the many research projects that uncovered the essential links between cigarette smoking and cancer, and also subsidized tobacco farmers and exporters of cigarettes to support domestic production of tobacco and to promote the overseas sale of cigarettes.

Against this mighty alliance, the anti-cancer forces were weak, unorganized, and financially insignificant. Their potential strength was the truth, and it would take time for the battle to become one between equals. In 1957 only a few scientists and physicians were prepared to serve as activists within the glare of the public arena.

The day after the big story broke in the New York *Times,* I got a message from the manager of the Tex McCrary television show (the big nighttime talk show at that time), asking me to appear on the program to present the point of view of the study group. Clearance was received from the American Cancer Society, and arrangements were made for the time and place of the interview. I was instructed to wear a blue shirt and was told that no one else would be there to present any opposing views. My younger son, Robby (three years old at the time), offered to lend me his holster and guns, because in his experience with television, this was an essential part of one's costume. His instinct on how to handle the media turned out to be quite accurate.

My chance to present the findings of the study group to a large audience proved to be illusory. Shortly before midnight, the manager of the show called again, this time to inform me that the invitation had been withdrawn. He was apologetic, but businesslike: "The network wouldn't permit you to go on. It is, after all, understandable—the tobacco industry has a large investment in television advertising." To soften his rejection, he offered to arrange for a radio interview in the near future. It, of course, never materialized.

My first reaction to this reversal was relief—this would have been my first television appearance and I was a bit nervous as well as doubtful of my ability to do justice to the subject.

By morning, however, anger had replaced relief. I became indignant at the high-handedness with which this vital health information was being kept from the public. After conferring with officials at the American Cancer Society, it was agreed that I send a letter of protest exposing this episode to the New York *Times*. In the letter, I related the circumstances of the invitation and the cancellation and concluded that the issue of arbitrary censorship in matters of serious health concern to the public overrode the issue of whether cigarette smoking caused lung cancer. I also quoted verbatim the words of the manager of the show.

Val Adams, the television reporter for the *Times,* requested permission to use this information in a news story. I acquiesced, assuming that the full contents and the exact wording of the rejection would be reported. I was mistaken. A day later, the story appeared—but my accusation wasn't the central focus; Tex McCrary's denial and explanation were. The impression created was that my invitation had been conditional upon the ability of Mr. McCrary to secure an adequate representative of the opposite point of view. He was unable, he claimed, to find a single scientist or physician in the entire United States willing to present the other side. It obviously would not have been fair, therefore, to permit me to appear, alone and unopposed. It would have been un-American.

On the following Sunday, Jack Gould, television editor of the *Times,* wrote a feature article in the News of the Week in Review section titled "Busy Big Brother." He cited this incident as an example of how the television industry used the technique of equal time to studiously avoid the presentation of those controversial subjects that might incur the wrath of their clients, the advertisers.

I had written to the *Times* requesting that they publish my letter in full. Their response was that the subject already had been covered in a news article; therefore it would be repetitive to publish the letter. By this act, the New York *Times* avoided publishing the statement made by the manager of the program to me giving the reason for the cancellation.

Many of the national newsweeklies carried the story; things were getting hot. An invitation arrived from a new experimental program on a local TV station. I was told that this was to be a program in which the interviewer would act as devil's advocate. I thought this was fine, and in my anxiety to penetrate the tobacco industry's imposed TV blackout, I accepted. The flamboyant title of the show, "Experiment X," should have aroused my suspicions and made me more circumspect.

On the day prior to the broadcast, I was somewhat startled to read in the television section of the *Daily News* that the interviewer would be wearing a black mask in order to retain his anonymity throughout the program. Furthermore, he would make a determined effort to provoke me into walking "offstage" in the midst of the discussion. This format was clearly designed to prevent any meaningful discussion of the facts. My initial (and angry) reaction was to disengage from the whole thing, but I soon realized that the TV establishment could distort my withdrawal and announce that a leading member of the National Study Group on Smoking and Health had been offered his day in court but "chickened out." They could then use this as evidence to prove there was no censorship on television. It was obvious that I had been rather cleverly mousetrapped.

The only remaining choice was to fulfill the commitment and attempt a dignified, lucid, and convincing presentation of the subject. The belief that this was even remotely possible proved to be as ludicrous as my innocent and eager acceptance of the original invitation.

In the remaining hours, my apprehension continued to mount,

and just before broadcast time approached, I was in a state of panic, especially when, in the television studio, I was suddenly confronted by a huge torso with a head, face, neck, and upper shoulders completely covered by a black hood containing small slits for the eyes, nose, and mouth. This figure sitting squarely opposite me—on a raised podium behind a table—stared directly at me through those slits in the hood and never broke his silence. Meanwhile, the crew of engineers and cameramen had set up cameras and hot glaring lights—all focused directly toward me.

In the few seconds remaining before the opening of the broadcast, I was afraid that, at my initial attempt to speak, an inaudible squeak would emerge from my vocal cords. In order to allay this fear and the paralyzing tension, I forced myself to make some insignificant pleasantries to the mysterious moderator, but he neither replied nor made any gesture of acknowledgement. He continued his direct stare and maintained an unbroken silence.

Then we were on the air. A booming voice emerged from behind the hood: "Dr. Spain, are you aware of the following facts?" And with that, he waved aloft a sheaf of documents and papers from which he "quoted" names of many scientists along with considerable evidence discrediting the conclusions of the study group. At the end of this introductory tirade, he challenged me. "Well, what have you got to say to all of this?"

Somehow I contained myself, and audible words did issue from my lips. I managed to keep to my prepared plan for this presentation, despite a barrage of disruptive comments from my host. While proceeding with this account of the report linking cigarette smoking to lung cancer, I was bothered by the peculiar sensation that my voice had taken on an independent existence, out of reach of my control and thoughts. To me, as an observer of my own voice, it did not sound at all convincing. On one occasion my inquisitor shouted (as if he were the invited guest): "You're not giving me an equal share of the time."

At last it was over—and I felt both relieved and frustrated. The unknown hatchetman now stripped off his hood and revealed himself. It was Victor Lasky, who at that time was unknown to me. After talking to him, I felt that he had considered the interview a contest of wits. He invited me to have a drink with him. Hiding my disgust, I had a quick one, excused myself, and hurried off. The television industry could now record another proud episode in its distinguished history of rendering service to the public. After all, despite the pressure of its benefactors, TV had given a fair hearing to an important health matter.

Subsequently I learned of many similar acts of censorship. In one instance a panel of prominent physicians had taped a discussion on cancer prevention. When the tape was broadcast, all of their remarks on the hazards of smoking had been carefully edited out—without their knowledge or consent. They complained but never received a satisfactory explanation. On another occasion a major scientific medical society—paying for its own time on television—was forced to delete any comments pertaining to cigarette smoking and lung cancer. The orders had come from the top.

But time was beginning to work in our favor, and several years later I was asked by John Osmondson, at the time a science writer for the New York *Times,* to appear with him for a discussion of practical means of curtailing the smoking habit. This was still in the earlier days of the breakthrough, so it was on New York City's educational station, Channel 13 (NET).

I took advantage of this appearance to achieve something that until then I had failed to accomplish. It had never seemed appropriate to me that hospitals, institutions caring for the sick and supposedly concerned with the prevention of disease, should aid and abet the promotion of cancer by allowing cigarette vending machines to be installed in their facilities. All my efforts to have them removed from my own, Brookdale Hospital, had been rebuffed. As far as I knew, this situation prevailed in all hospitals. It was merely a matter of administrative apathy.

With this television broadcast in the offing, I went to the hospital administrator and offered him a chance to have Brookdale Hospital mentioned. This was a chance for some publicity, so he consented. John Osmondson, during the discussion, asked what immediate practical steps could be taken by physicians and hospitals to curb the smoking habit. I suggested that one small and practical educational step was to remove cigarette vending machines from all health facilities—as had been done, for example, at Brookdale Hospital. I added that a sign could also be erected at the vacated spot that might read, "Here once stood a cigarette vending machine, removed to halt the spread of lung cancer and other diseases." Many hospitals and health facilities have since followed suit. At many large medical conventions, ash trays are no longer supplied in the meeting rooms, and as many as one hundred thousand physicians have modified their smoking habits.

Organized medicine has little to boast of concerning its role in this campaign, however. Individual doctors, too, have been slow to react on this issue. I became keenly aware of this when *CA, A Bulletin of Cancer Progress,* published by the American Cancer Society, requested that I prepare an article on the duty of the physician toward his patients in regard to cigarette smoking. This was in 1959, and at that time physicians' attitudes were mainly conditioned by the quality and relevance of their education in medical school. Their outlook on patient care was formed by the pressure to specialize. Extreme specialization has been an unfortunate by-product of the rapid growth of medical knowledge, leading to a fragmentation of medical practice in which the physician views the patient mainly as an organ or a disease and not as a total human being with a past, present, and future. This, too often, causes the doctor to relate exclusively to the illness rather than to the person. It is this failure to comprehend health in a dynamic, total, and historical perspective that partially inhibits concern about the welfare of the patient twenty or thirty years hence. The remoteness of an immediate act of prevention from the potential benefit to be derived many years in the future is one of the difficulties.

Medical-school training, reinforced by the attitudes and pressures generated from a laissez-faire system of competitive medicine, is geared to the "quick result" and the "rapid pay-off," the prompt, discernible, and tangible effect. In any action designed to prevent cancer of the lung from developing in an interval of twenty-five years, there is no close or direct personal feeling of accomplishment for the doctor, who probably won't be there to see his good deed have its effect. The difficulty arises from the contrast between the positive actions a doctor is used to—giving injections, ordering medicines, operating in the treatment of an acute illness—and the negative action required by the problem of smoking, that of taking something away from a patient in order to prevent the possible development of a future sickness. For this reason, preventive medicine in the area of cigarette smoking is not readily applied by the physician and even less readily appreciated and accepted by the patient.

Surely the physician should spend at least as much time informing and advising his patients of the dangers of smoking as he does in administering transfusions and stimulants in order to prolong life for a few agonizing hours or days in terminal or inoperable cancer cases. Unquestionably, these efforts would eventually prove to be more rewarding. If any small fraction of general practitioners, alone in their offices and with no fancy equipment, would devote the time and effort needed to convince a few of their younger adult patients not to begin smoking or to break the habit, more meaningful and useful man-hours of life would be preserved than all that heart transplants (with the attendant expense and ballyhoo) could produce in the foreseeable future.

One must contend with the resistance of even some eminent physicians. We have all heard of the well-known British doctor (a smoker) who became irritated at all the articles he read about smoking, and so gave up reading. A popular internist in my home town, who was noted for his large clientele (consisting of society ladies) once publicly referred to my anti-smoking efforts as "neurotic." "After all," he said, "there is no evidence to support the thesis that smoking is dangerous. And we all know that cancer is emotional in origin anyway." In a later discussion with him, I learned that he had never read a single word of the Surgeon General's report on the subject.

For doctors to tell others not to smoke, they must first set the pattern themselves. "The only rational way of educating is to be an example," said Albert Einstein. "If one can't help it, a warning example." It makes my hackles rise to hear patients say: "My doctor is a regular guy: he lets me do anything I want."

The American Medical Association, which should have been the motivating force in educating the public and the prime mover for legislative controls, was the last of all major medical organizations to take a definitive and forthright stand. Belatedly, in December 1968, the AMA finally urged its members to "take a strong stand against smoking by any means at their command." This was many years after all the hard evidence had been collected and long after all the other notable scientific medical organizations had made official statements and initiated educational campaigns on the hazards of smoking. Could this procrastination have been partially the result of a $10 million gift given to the AMA research fund by the Tobacco Industry Research Committee (TIRC)? Perhaps the delay had been influenced by the rumored logrolling deal between the representatives and senators from tobacco-producing states and the AMA's legislative apparatus, in which the AMA agreed not to press for legislative controls of cigarette advertising in return for support in preventing governmental intrusion into medical practice. These same tobacco-state congressmen succeeded in blocking, for at least a year, an appropriation recommended by the President's advisers: it was to go to the Public Health Service and be used to inform the public of the danger of smoking; they also forced the PHS not to display specially prepared educational anti-smoking posters.

The behavior of a small number of scientists has been open to question as well. One can only speculate at the underlying motivation of a former university president and director of a famous research laboratory who in 1944, as managing director of the American Cancer Society, could state: ". . . it would seem unwise to fill the lungs repeatedly with a suspension of fine particles of tobacco products of which smoke consists. It is difficult to see how such particles can be prevented from being lodged in the lungs and when so located, how they can avoid producing a certain amount of irritation";* and then, in 1966, in his newer capacity as scientific director of The Council for Tobacco Research (a tobacco-industry-financed fund) could make the following statement in his annual report: "In the 1964–65 Report it was mentioned that over the years experimental and clinical evidence to support the thesis that cigarette smoking exercises a direct carcinogenic effect on man has not been forthcoming. After reviewing another year of research, this statement still expresses the state of our scientific knowledge."† A man may modify his opinion, but this change, given the evidence of the Surgeon General's report, seems absurd. One would like to believe his new opinion was based on ignorance or on misinterpretation, but there seems to me to be a less forgivable reason—a change of masters.

A prime example of the way the tobacco industry treats the public's health needs was provided by Mr. John F. Gillespie, director of the New York State Tobacco Distributors' Association, in a hearing before the New York State Senate Special Committee on Smoking and Health. He was asking for a delay in any action regarding cigarettes on the part of the state legislature, stating that the implementation of controls would lead to "irreparable repercussions in practically every facet of our industrial fabric." He finished his remarks with a jibe at his opponents: "And now I want to point out there are several gentlemen here, like our good President, John Ludlow [of the Tobacco Distributors' Association], who have no need to fear lung cancer, because several very eminent doctors have pointed out that people who are bald do not ever get lung cancer. Now, these statistics are just as factual, my dear friends, as is the

* Quoted by Harold S. Diehl, in *Tobacco and Your Health*, McGraw-Hill, 1969, pp. 21–22.

† *Report of the Scientific Director*, The Council for Tobacco Research, 1966.

statistical report of those 'ten boys' down in Washington known as the Surgeon General's committee."‡

I, of course, was one of the boys. Among other scientists to whom he referred were the dean of the Yale School of Medicine, the professor of statistics at Harvard University, the chairman of the Department of Pathology at the University of Pittsburgh, the former editor-in-chief of *Cancer Research,* the chairman of the Department of Medicine at the University of Indiana. The other four were of the same stature.

Mr. Gillespie's statement was a small part of the sudden relentless and vicious counterattack by the tobacco industry. The country was flooded with subsidized paperback books and magazine articles aimed at denigrating and confusing this important scientific breakthrough. *Barron's National Business and Financial Weekly,* in an article, referred to those who were working on this health problem as "witch doctors." Another report, in the *National Enquirer,* was captioned "Most Medical Experts Say Cigarette Cancer Link Is Bunk—70,000,000 Smokers Falsely Alarmed."

The unremitting propaganda and much more led Emerson Foote, president of one of the largest advertising firms in this country, to resign from his company. In doing so he said, "Basically, the promotion of cigarette smoking is a clear application of the principle of the primacy of profits over people. . . ." He was one of the exceptional few who had the humanity to escape the corrosive effects on the human spirit of the Madison Avenue jungle.

But interview after interview with habitual adult smokers has convinced me that, ultimately, habit will remain the most difficult barrier to overcome in the anti-cancer endeavor. In Dr. Wynder's laboratory, technicians paint cigarette-tar extracts

‡ *Report of the Senate Special Committee on Smoking and Health,* no. 77, 1964, p. 22.

daily on the skins of thousands of mice and watch the cancers growing. They continue to do this with a lighted cigarette in one hand and the little paintbrush in the other.

This kind of triumph of blind compulsion over reason was vividly depicted by a thirty-five-year-old man who was smoking three packs a day. He was a participant in a study I was conducting on the factors in our environment that might increase the risk of heart attacks. His son was twelve and his daughter was ten. The excessively heavy smoking habit caught my attention, and I decided to spend some time with him. He explained away this extreme habit by stating that he was willing to pay the price for the pleasure he derived from smoking. I acquainted him with the fact that at his present rate of smoking, he would have a better than one out of ten chance of dying from lung cancer before he was fifty, as compared to the non-smoker, who would only have one chance out of two hundred and fifty at a comparable age. I reminded him that in twelve years his daughter would be graduating from college and his son would just be getting married, and he would more likely be bedridden, gasping his last gasp and coughing his last cough. It would be little comfort to him, the dying father, to say to his wife and children: "Don't weep over me—I'm merely paying the price for years of indulgence in a so-called pleasurable habit."

Hardly had I finished depicting this deathbed scene when he reached into his pocket, pulled out a pack of cigarettes, crushed it in his clenched hand and then tore the pack to shreds. After thanking me, he got up, walked into the adjoining waiting lounge and asked the first person he saw for a cigarette. He could not have realized what he was doing. It was blind compulsion triumphing over reason.

That is why the major point of attack must be on the adolescent, the teen-ager, the presmoker, and the one who has just begun. In them the habit is either absent or not yet well established. To achieve meaningful, lasting, and optimum results in this group, the health advisers, physicians, and teachers must probe to find out why young people want to smoke. They must have insight themselves into the problem and be prepared to deal with the issue not as a moral question but as a problem of health and survival, pure and simple. They should be prepared to help the young destroy false idols and motivations for smoking—the kind that adolescents are so susceptible to, such as being a part of the crowd, or looking sophisticated or "with it." The young must be made to overcome their lack of identification with those over forty who develop cancer— because someday, that could be them. And if all the communications media cease presenting cigarette smoking as a desirable activity and use their persuasiveness to show that it is no more than an ugly form of personal air pollution, significant inroads can be made in the lung-cancer toll. The banning of cigarette advertising from television is only one small step in the right direction, since manufacturers have simply switched their advertising to other media; by May 1971, cigarette advertising in magazines, for example, had doubled since the TV ban went into effect. A lot of people seem to think the danger went away with the ads.

Despite the staggering evidence reported annually by the Surgeon General, despite the total ban on cigarette promotion on television, more women are now smoking greater quantities of cigarettes than at any time in the past ten years. This unfortunate step toward equality with men has also begun to equalize men and women in the health area: associated with this rise in smoking among women (according to recent research statistics of my own) is a heightened risk of dying suddenly at a younger age from heart attacks, and an increased chance of developing pulmonary emphysema (overdistended lungs).

Two current myths on smoking ought to be dispelled: Advocates of the legalization of marijuana claim that the smoking of grass is not cancer-producing. To the contrary, recent studies indicate that smoking of five joints a day, with the holding of each puff in the lungs ten seconds, has the equivalent adverse effect on the lungs as smoking more than a pack of cigarettes. The cancer-producing tars are also present in marijuana smoke. The other illusion is that a safe cigarette will soon appear on the market. Less hazardous cigarettes are already available, and perhaps better ones will be forthcoming—but there isn't a truly cancer-proof cigarette, and there won't be in the foreseeable future. Inherent in the burning process of all vegetable matter (lettuce, spinach, or tobacco) is the production of cancer-producing tars. The amount of cancer-causing substances in the tar may vary from one product to another, but significant quantities are always present. The amount of tar can be reduced by changing the speed and temperature of the burning process, but then the cigarette will not burn smoothly or feel cool and of course will not be competitive in the market place. For more than a decade, much research with vast expenditures has gone into this project, with few tangible or practical results. To a certain extent, a cigarette becomes less harmful; to that extent, of course, it is a step forward. But to think of a safe smoke at present is a pipe dream.

Paradoxically it may be the non-smokers, potentially the largest protest group in the country, rather than the smokers, who may eventually turn the tide. Ever since early 1972, when the Surgeon General reported on the harmful effects of the smoke from nearby smokers on non-smokers, the abstainer's attitude has become more hostile toward the addict. The non-smokers are now organizing into militant and activist groups demanding complete protection in all public places from the smoke of smokers. The slogans on their anti-smoking posters reflect this change. Whereas they formerly read, PLEASE DON'T SMOKE, PEOPLE ARE BREATHING, they now read, PLEASE DON'T BREATHE, PEOPLE ARE SMOKING.

2. CURES CAN KILL

Modern technology . . . with one hand is the friend of man, and with the other strikes him down.

C. P. Snow

The diseases of the past have little in common with the diseases of the present, save that we die of them.

Agnes Repplier

Any rational individual will agree that, on the whole, modern medical practices have done vastly more good than harm. Nevertheless some patients do die from their cures, and as a result, the good physician will keep in mind this cardinal rule, ancient even in the time of Hippocrates: "Primum non nocere"—first do no harm. I have written a textbook for the medical profession on this subject of doctor-induced diseases and have also lectured on it before many medical societies in various parts of the country. It was therefore inevitable that sooner or later I would be called upon to testify as an expert witness in a trial involving the adverse effects of medical treatment. When the time came to appear in court, it was a big case concerned with a basic legal issue of liability, and the financial stakes were high.

Ironically I found myself on the side of the defendant, the gigantic international XYZ Chemical Corporation, and not, as I would have expected, on the side of the plaintiff, Ms. Winifred Gedney. She was allegedly harmed by the drug named Procidin, manufactured by the XYZ company. Yet, in this instance, XYZ was the more logical of the two adversaries for me to be involved with.

The stringent regulations recently adopted by the Food and Drug Administration for the control of medicaments manufactured by the chemical and pharmaceutical companies have only partially stemmed the introduction of large numbers of new drugs each year. The market continues to be flooded, and the average doctor is overwhelmed in his attempt to remain abreast of the new information on the drugs he learned about in his earlier years of training, let alone the new drugs.

All drugs are chemicals, and thus are potentially harmful. Pertinent to the XYZ case was the question of whether a harmful reaction was known to the drug company, based on its own studies during the developmental and testing phase of the drug. If so, had this information been immediately and widely disseminated to the regulatory agencies and to the medical profession? If complications from the use of this medication appeared much later, after the drug had been in clinical use for some time, did the company take adequate steps to send out proper warnings on the newly uncovered, dangerous aspects of the drug?

The suit was brought against the XYZ Chemical Corporation when Winifred Gedney, who had been using Procidin* for several months, developed a lung condition for which she was hospitalized. The physician in charge of the case in the hospital blamed her lung problem on the prolonged use of Pro-

* A fictitious name for the real drug.

cidin. He discontinued the use of this medication, and her condition began to clear. This was the point at which the attorney representing the XYZ company consulted me.

There were several questions the defense attorney wanted me to clarify. Besides a chronic infection of Ms. Gedney's bladder, for which Procidin had been prescribed, she also suffered from arthritis. Rheumatism can become complicated by a lung disorder. Can arthritis also be accompanied by lung complications? Could Ms. Gedney's lung condition have been caused by the arthritis rather than by the drug? Does the lung disease caused by the drug resemble the lung complication associated with arthritis, and if so, is it possible to distinguish between the two? It was because of my experience with lung diseases, and also because I had testified in a prior hearing on these same two questions (but then on the side of the plaintiff), that I had been retained in this case. In the prior hearing, I had maintained that the changes in the lung produced by arthritis and by the drug were so similar that it was virtually impossible to tell them apart with any degree of certainty. The only possible way was to wait and see what happened after the drug had been discontinued. If the process cleared up without any additional treatment, the drug was probably the cause of the problem. I repeated this view to the attorney for XYZ, and I also offered the opinion in court during Ms. Gedney's case.

So far in this matter I was of very little help to my client. Crucial to the outcome of this litigation was the doctrine of liability. The authoritative American Law Institute recently, in its restatement of the law of torts, added some comments about how liability applies to drugs. It said: "An absence of significant directions or warnings can render a product defective under the doctrine. Unavoidably unsafe products such as the vaccine used for Pasteur treatment of rabies, or new and experimental drugs, are not defective if properly prepared and accompanied by proper directions and warnings."†

My analysis of the directions and warnings as to the possible adverse effects of Procidin indicated that the XYZ company had been diligent and proper in these areas. When isolated reports of the pulmonary complications arising from the prolonged use of Procidin came to the attention of their medical department, they investigated them and reported all the events in an article published in the *New England Journal of Medicine*, a leading publication read by many physicians. They also printed the warning in the literature and brochures accompanying the drug. The admonitions were also included in the Physicians Desk Reference. This is the doctor's drug bible, which he consults or should consult to familiarize himself with a drug and its possible harmful effects before he prescribes it for a patient. I did not find the drug company derelict.

In reviewing the history of the case and the care that Winifred Gedney received, I became convinced that her original physician was the real culprit. This doctor had given the drug to the plaintiff, had renewed its use over the telephone without another examination, and had failed to heed the early signs of the beginnings of the pulmonary disorder. According to my way of thinking and the law on liability as I understood it, the doctor should have been named the defendant and not the XYZ Chemical Corporation.

But the plaintiff's lawyer had an advantage. He didn't care who was really negligent in this case; he was concerned only with winning as large a financial award as he could for his client. The trial was in a rural town. Everyone knew and liked Winifred Gedney's doctor. The lawyer sensed he could never get a local jury to convict the doctor of malpractice. On the

† Sec. 402A, *Legal Medicine Annual, 1970,* Cyril Wecht, ed., Appleton-Century-Crofts.

other hand, the XYZ company was located in another state. It was large, rich, and impersonal. It was logical to attack it. This he did, and despite evidence to the contrary and my expert testimony, he won the case and received a substantial award for his client. By this time, she had fully recovered from the pulmonary disorder, which I feel was never clearly proved to be caused by Procidin, as she was treated with cortisone after the Procidin was stopped.

As the Food and Drug Administration has become more attentive to the claims the pharmaceutical houses make for their products, the manufacturers have become more cautious and meticulous in their statements and warnings. This has shifted responsibility for adverse drug risks to the physicians, some of whom fail to heed the manufacturers' warnings and are negligent in watching their patients for early signs of harmful drug reactions. In the future, more of the legal actions will be directed against the doctors and fewer against the manufacturers.

A decade before I testified in the XYZ case, I had already become aware that the environment of the patient was daily growing more complicated. Each year, the potency and number of drugs, as well as the number and variety of other diagnostic and therapeutic agents and devices, increases at a rate that, if it does not defy comprehension, at least challenges the individual doctor's ability to digest their significance and modes of action. The tools and products that have contributed to medical progress in the past decade are unprecedented in the history of mankind, but these tools are two-edged swords. In one large hospital at any given moment, fifty out of every one thousand beds are constantly occupied by the victims of complications from various therapeutic agents. And this does not account for the beds occupied by the victims of the complications from diagnostic and therapeutic instrumentation. One author has called both these types of complications "diseases of medical progress." Iatrogenic disease (originating with the doctor: iatro—doctor; genesis—origin) can now take its place almost as an equal alongside bacteria as an important factor in the development of human illness.

The dual nature of the medicines doctors prescribe is akin to the split behavior of Dr. Jekyll and Mr. Hyde. In Robert Louis Stevenson's story, Jekyll, a responsible physician, discovers a powder that transforms him into a base creature (Mr. Hyde). For a while, he is able to control this metamorphosis. But Hyde's wild lusts prove to be insatiable, and the doctor loses control.

How do we go about detecting and uncovering the culprits that cause iatrogenic diseases? Tracking down Hyde can be a complex, prolonged, tedious, and at times fruitless task. All the skills and techniques of the relentless detective are required. Everything in the past and present of the patient's medical environment must be considered suspect.

It is often difficult to get a handle on the case and to know where to begin. The answer rarely comes from some brilliant intuitive stroke of luck; rather, it is derived from painstaking investigation into every aspect of the case and, as such, requires thorough understanding of the patient, his illnesses past and present, his eating habits, his occupation, and even where he lives and travels. Intelligent interviewing techniques must discover all that has been done to him medically for a good portion of his life. Any case under study must be compared with similar, isolated cases and with those compiled in the official central agencies that register harmful reactions to various drugs.

A good example is the case of the twelve-year-old boy whom I autopsied about fifteen years ago. I found his bones, liver, and lungs to be riddled with cancer. These tumor invasions had spread throughout his body from a malignant growth that I found to be originating in his thyroid gland (the thyroid gland is situated in the neck, overlying the main windpipe, and it partly controls the metabolism of the body). Usually, thyroid cancer is not found in young people, and in prior years I would merely have regarded this finding in a youth as an unexplained curiosity. Personal experience and a reading of the current medical reports, however, had diminished my surprise at this occurrence. Doctors, in the years immediately preceding this autopsy, had witnessed a significant increase in the number of youths harboring thyroid cancers. The explanation for this phenomenon, puzzling at first, was soon discovered and was well publicized by the time I had made my examination.

So now I was almost positive that I knew the cause of this boy's cancer. It would be nailed down as soon as I could question the dead boy's parents. My guess proved to be right. The father, after some thought, recalled that their family doctor, during a routine examination of the boy as an infant, had found what he thought to be an enlarged thymic gland (an organ situated within the upper portion of the chest, next to the thyroid gland). During those years, a widespread theory prevailed that enlarged thymic glands were the cause of sudden unexplained deaths (still called "crib deaths") in otherwise healthy infants. The enlarged thymic gland was thought to press on the adjacent heart or windpipe, fatally injuring the infants. The recommended cure was a massive dose of X rays to shrink the enlarged gland. The young boy had received X-ray treatments on the lower region of his neck and the upper part of his chest.

There was a lack of awareness by most doctors—including this boy's—that the cells of an infant's thyroid gland are especially vulnerable to the effects of X rays and that a late consequence of damage to these cells could be cancer. The thyroid gland is a neighbor of the thymus, and some infants receiving X-ray treatments for the reasons mentioned eventually developed cancer, which showed up five to ten years later. This young boy was one of these unfortunates; he had been given cancer by his family doctor's treatment.

The thymic theory of crib deaths has since been disproved, and the X-ray treatment has long since been abandoned. In this instance, the solution of what was causing cancer, and the realization that X rays were the culprits, came to light because a few medical investigators had done some excellent detective work. They had approached the problem exactly as a criminologist does, grouping together the clues in similar cases: the ages of the victims, the "locales" of the crimes, the presence of "fingerprints" or telltale marks that would identify the common denominators.

When these youthful cases of thyroid cancers appeared, the various institutions seeing them pooled their information and engaged in a co-operative analysis of the features of each case. The first lead uncovered was that the cancers occurred equally in boys and girls. This clue was important, because the even sex ratio differed from the distribution in the more common form of adult thyroid cancer, which is predominant in women. This meant that the cause of the new cancers in the young might be different from that in the adult, because in the young the culprit must have similar access to males and females.

Turning to the national data bank on thyroid cancer for the profile of these cases, investigators noted that most occurred between the ages of five and fifteen. Long experience with other forms of human cancer and with experimental studies in animals had shown that it takes approximately from five to ten years, more or less, for a cancer to grow to a degree that it becomes obvious to the examining doctor. This placed the time of the original exposure to the offending agent between infancy and about five or six years of age. Next came a visit to the rogues' gallery (cancer registry), where information had been accumulated over the years on the best-known and established causes of human cancer. From these files, two of the most likely suspects, radiation and hormones, were selected for further investigation. Either of these could have been given 1) to the mother while she was pregnant or 2) directly to the young infant. Suspect number one, radiation, had a long history of previous crimes, having produced cancer of the bone in radium-dial watch workers, cancer of the skin in individuals who had previously been radiated for sundry skin disorders years before, and an increasing number of malignant tumors in the survivors of the Hiroshima bombing. Armed with this information, the investigators returned to the best material witnesses, the parents, who were specifically asked if their children had been exposed at any time between infancy and the age of five to X rays and whether they had ever received any form of hormone treatment. This was the pay-off, because the sum of the answers revealed that 90–100 per cent of the children developing this form of thyroid cancer had been treated with X rays to the region of the neck or upper chest at a young age. In addition to this indication of X-ray treatments, it was learned that some physicians had also been X-raying enlarged tonsils in order to shrink them down. This was usually done in children closer to the age of five and accounted for the somewhat older cases, occurring around the age of fifteen. Conclusive evidence incriminating the X rays came when this form of treatment in the young was discontinued and the rising frequency of these cancers was reversed.

More subtle than this case was the explanation for the tragic and sudden death of a nineteen-year-old black woman while undergoing a tooth extraction in the dental chair. Prior to autopsy, I talked to the dentist. The dentist informed me that he had anesthetized the patient with nitrous oxide, commonly known as "laughing gas." It was regarded as a mild and reasonably safe anesthetic and was routinely used years ago by many dentists. The dose of gas given did not appear excessive.

The autopsy at first failed to explain the fatality, and I was forced to temporarily list the cause of the expiration on the death certificate as "undetermined pending chemical and microscopic examination." Sometimes, further study fails to clear up the reasons for death, but, this time, examination of the brain tissue solved the case. Looking at the brain through the microscope, I could see that almost every small artery, and many of the tiny capillaries that transport blood, were stuffed with adherent and deformed red blood cells, preventing the oxygen-carrying blood from reaching the vital areas. The woman, unbeknown to the dentist (and most likely to herself as well), had a mild and symptomless form of a condition known as sickle-cell disease. This is an inherited disorder of the chemical structure of the red blood corpuscles, present in about 10 per cent of the black population, which makes the cells extremely vulnerable to a lack of oxygen. When deprived of oxygen, the normally round, disklike cells become elongated and resemble small sickles. This causes them to stick to each other, forming plugs in the channels of the small blood vessels. Nitrous oxide, when properly used, is relatively harmless in the "normal" person but can be exceedingly dangerous in the sickle-cell patient because of this anesthetic's ability to deplete the blood's oxygen supply. Nowadays a screening test is widely used to detect the hidden or unknown carriers of this defect so that proper precautions can be taken if people having it should require anesthesia. If the dentist had been aware of this potential problem (as he should have been), he could have questioned the woman concerning this condition and, to avoid the pitfall, used another form of anesthesia.

Three hundred years ago, the renowned playwright Molière observed: "Almost all men die of their medicines, not their diseases." Deaths and disorders caused by doctors have been with us since ancient times, but never in the volume that exists today. In present circumstances it is hard for a doctor to resist becoming "drug-happy." Thousands of new medicines pour off the chemical assembly line and erupt with great fanfare on the market. Pharmaceutical companies, in intense competition with each other for a larger share of the market, bombard the physicians with a glittering supply of drug samples. Slick and expensively put together magazines, house newspapers, and sophisticated and attractive brochures flood the doctors' mailboxes. Young interns and residents are seduced by drug houses extending free invitations to dinner at the best local steak houses and by gifts of instruments, flashlights, and other mechanical gadgets. Supersalesmen known as "detail men" roam the country and get into every doctor's office to recite recently rehearsed sales pitches from their repertoire glorifying the curative merits and safety of each new drug. Specially prepared educational films on a myriad of medical subjects are loaned to the hospitals for teaching conferences, and of course, within the context of these films their special products are promoted. At every major national or state medical convention, the exhibit hall is filled with costly, glittering, and overwhelming pharmaceutical displays, always extolling the incomparable curative virtues of their wares; and at these exhibit counters, the wives of the physicians line up to get gifts of special soaps, powders, perfumes, etc.

Prior to the tightening of the Food and Drug Administration's code, many physicians were paid fat fees to perform so-called scientific tests on different drugs in their office practices so they could then give testimonials for advertising purposes. How many physicians could resist this, and for how long?

The Food and Drug Administration tightened up on the lax and inadequate testing and licensing procedures in 1960—only after the international Thalidomide disaster, when hundreds of infants were born with cruel deformities because the mothers had taken the drug during pregnancy (Thalidomide enjoyed widespread use, particularly in Germany, as a tranquilizer and for the relief of nausea in pregnant women though it was banned in the United States by the FDA). So many useless and dangerous drugs have been released for human consumption despite this tightening that in 1968 there were at least two thousand articles in the world medical literature reporting iatrogenic disorders; in 1969 it had risen to three thousand. And with it, of course, rose the number of autopsies my colleagues and I performed on the victims of fatal drug-induced complications.

Without question, antibiotics, primarily penicillin, are the most formidable weapons currently available in combating infection, but few medicines have produced as many iatrogenic illnesses as these same antibiotics. There are times when a doctor has no choice but to use them. It is also true that these antibacterial medicines are prescribed when there really is no clear need.

Those doctors who compulsively grab at each new drug almost the very day it is released for general use were the target of Dr. Isadore Snapper's satirical remarks at one of our weekly hospital-wide teaching conferences, when he expressed his attitude toward any new medication. Dr. Snapper, formerly director of medicine at Brookdale Hospital, and a clinician of international fame, said: "When a new drug is manufactured, for the first five years it should be experimented with on rats, dogs, and monkeys; the next five years on my enemies; the following five years on my relatives; and the last five years on my friends. By this time, I am sure that the drug will finally have proven to be useless and will be ready to be discarded, so I don't have to take it at all." This pointedly gross exaggeration, told in 1958, was nevertheless remarkably prophetic. Ten years later, an expert committee of the National Academy of

Sciences assigned to a drug-evaluation task by the FDA found that of three thousand drugs on the market and in constant use by physicians, only 25 per cent could be classified as effective, and even in the acceptable drugs these experts found it necessary to add a qualifying "but" to the "effective" classification of each of them.

A case in point illustrating the indiscriminate use of a "wonder drug" was the fatal misadventure that befell Dr. Charles Zimmer's son. It was with difficulty that I autopsied the ten-year-old boy. Charles Zimmer had been my close friend and classmate throughout undergraduate college and medical school and was at the time of his son's death a colleague of mine at Grasslands Hospital, in Westchester.

Only the night before, his son had had an acute attack of the "croup," an intense infection of the upper air passages accompanied by much swelling, which severely impedes the flow of air into and out of the lungs. This illness, sometimes serious and occasionally rapidly fatal, may require an on-the-spot tracheotomy (cutting directly into the windpipe through the neck to allow oxygen to enter directly into the lungs). Ironically Dr. Zimmer specializes in diseases of the throat and is an expert in the treatment of such an infection. He had saved the lives of many children with this affliction by his proper and urgent intervention. Dr. Zimmer promptly injected his son with penicillin and was in the act of rushing him to the hospital when the boy turned blue. Within a few minutes he was dead.

At the autopsy, there was clear evidence of an overwhelming and fatal form of allergic shock—an adverse reaction sometimes seen following injections of penicillin. But why in this case? This lethal complication usually does not develop unless the patient has been previously exposed to the drug. Dr. Zimmer had done what he thought was correct and safest for his son; he did not feel he had any reason to fear any ill effect from the antibiotic, because, according to his best recollection, the boy had never before been given penicillin.

As it turned out, he had had a previous exposure to penicillin two years before, when he had been inoculated with Salk polio vaccine. Dr. Zimmer, along with many other physicians, was not aware that the pharmaceutical manufacturer had added penicillin to the early batches of polio vaccine as an added precaution to minimize the chances of contamination. The practice was soon discontinued; but in the interim, some children had been needlessly—and what was worse, unknowingly—sensitized to penicillin.

Today's biggest problem of doctor-induced disease is the widespread transmission of the hepatitis virus via blood. In this nation alone, more than five million units of blood are transfused each year, and in some clinics, one out of every ten patients receives blood. The ready availability of preserved blood and the relative ease of administering it, along with the increased demand due to the advances in radical cancer and cardiovascular surgery, have produced a staggering increase in the number of transfusions. Unfortunately, however, a sizable proportion of this increase is due to the indiscriminate use of blood in cases where there is no clear indication for its need. This wasteful and sometimes harmful practice is derived from the physician's desire to play it safe: "It's right at hand, easy to get, so let's give it"—almost as if a tablespoon of some old-fashioned tonic or cod-liver oil were being dispensed. This drunken orgy of blood-giving has helped to speed the spread of hepatitis, which now has reached epidemic proportions. Some estimate 3 per cent of all transfusion recipients are infected with one form of the hepatitis virus, and this is believed to account for several thousand fatalities a year. Recognition of this danger has forced a more sober approach in the use of blood, and hospitals have set up watchdog transfusion com-

mittees to check on the real need for blood whenever it is ordered by the doctors in a non-urgent situation.

The hideous commercial concept of buying and selling human blood is quite monstrous. Bigotry, greed, and ignorance
assume a front-running role in the history of "traffic in human
blood," one of the more gruesome chapters in the annals of
iatrogenic disease.

Before the days of blood banks and the know-how of blood
preservation, patients were transfused by a person-to-person
hookup system that sucked out blood directly from the donor
and pumped it immediately into the adjacent recipient. Racism
often prevented the only available donor from being utilized,
because it would have been foolhardy in most places to try to
obtain consent from a white recipient in order to infuse him
with a black person's blood, even if needed to save his life.
With the advent of blood banks, preserved blood was at first
segregated into separate refrigerators for "white" blood and
for "black" blood. Preserved black blood was rarely transfused into a white. World War II led to a tremendous need
for blood and an expansion of blood banks, and with this came
a breakdown of this non-scientific and bigoted practice, at least
in those areas where racism was not so virulent. Blood banks
became a vital part of the medical scene.

Then some enterprising blood-bank experts, in union with a
few hospitals, spotted the chance for a tidy profit from the
blood-banking business. In New York City a well-known blood
expert in co-operation with the now extinct and formerly prestigious Post-Graduate Hospital, on lower Second Avenue, joined
in a most notorious endeavor. My acquaintance with this operation began one cold winter's day while walking up Second
Avenue from my residence to Bellevue Hospital. I noticed a
long line of men waiting to enter a rather nondescript store.
My attention was directed to this scene because some of the

men had crutches, others had casts on their arms or legs, and most were thinly and shabbily clad. As I approached the group, I saw they were haggard and bore the characteristic features of the chronic alcoholic who has been living a long time on the Bowery. Curious as to why they had gathered here, away from their usual territory, I asked one of them what they were lined up for. I learned that the storefront was the entrance to a donor's center for a blood bank and that these men were waiting to sell their blood. This was in the winter of 1946, and the prevailing price paid to each for a pint of blood was five dollars. These were the same men, often encountered on the street, who begged, stole, and engaged in occasional odd jobs to secure sufficient funds to finance their alcoholic needs. In a sense, the plight of these men was similar to the current heroin addict who begs and steals to raise funds for his daily fix.

Intrigued by this, I decided to wait around and speak to some of the men who had already sold their blood and exited from the blood center. Most of them immediately rushed across the street to the nearest bar with their recent earnings to satisfy their craving for whiskey. I managed to engage one of them in conversation, and he told me that he sold his blood as often as five or six times a month. I wondered how this was possible, because it was the policy in most blood centers to accept no more than one pint of blood a month from any single individual. He told me this was no problem, because he made the rounds of several blood banks and never told them the truth as to when he had last given blood. I am sure these blood banks were aware of this practice, but in their own self-interest closed their eyes to it. The nurses or doctors at these centers never obtained a truthful or accurate history concerning whether these donors might recently have had jaundice and might still be harboring the hepatitis virus. If all this information were uncovered, it would have made their blood unacceptable. To make matters worse, these usually malnourished, sick, and sometimes disease-ridden alcoholics often developed an anemia caused by the excessive bloodletting. The anemia weakened some of them to the extent that they were admitted to Bellevue Hospital, where they in turn became the recipients of banked blood transfusions. This became commonplace enough for one of the Bellevue physicians to report a series of these instances in the *New York State Journal of Medicine,* in an article called "Blood Donor's Anemia."

The Post-Graduate Blood Bank Corporation paid $5.00 for a pint of blood and expended approximately $2.50 for processing. A pint of blood, at a total cost of $7.50, was sold to the participating hospitals for $15. The hospitals in turn billed patients $25. The annual estimated profits for this sole enterprise was well over one million dollars. An important key to this profitable venture was a cheap and ready source of raw material: human blood. The managers of the project displayed their ingenuity by posting signs advertising their offer to buy blood at $5.00 a pint in various employment agencies, exploiting the unemployed's immediate and desperate need for money.

Needless to say, banks of this sort were and are not entirely representative of what goes on in this field. Many hospitals and independent blood banks such as the Red Cross and the New York Blood Bank obtain, process, and distribute blood by strictly moral, medically sound, and humane methods, but the existence of even one unscrupulous operation is one too many.

In England, the practice of selling and buying human blood is looked upon as a monstrous act. No such thing exists there, and the frequency of transfusion-induced viral hepatitis is much lower than here. The U. S. Government has finally but belatedly taken cognizance of the harmful practice and has set about to regulate strictly the operation of blood banks.

Technology, as well as chemistry, has become the physician's master instead of his tool. A rather horrifying and inhuman example is the story of an eighty-four-year-old man who suffered cardiac arrest at a hospital that shall go nameless. The special bell system for alerting the Resuscitation and Cardiac Arrest team brought nurses and doctors running to the patient's bedside. The patient had a history of four previous severe heart attacks, and for the past three weeks had been barely kept alive. He was in a constant state of breathlessness and pain, flat in bed, hooked to all sorts of tubes and wires. He had told me that all he wanted was to die.

Within minutes, the team had assembled beside the man's bed. Each knew his assignment well. Swiftly and silently, without missing a beat, they went to the business at hand. One attached electrical apparatus to the patient. Another introduced a catheter into a vein. A third placed a tube into the patient's mouth and down his throat, and the fourth, a vigorous young surgical resident, jumped onto the bed, climbed astride the lifeless man, and began to apply external cardiac massage in an attempt to awaken the stilled heart. In his overexuberance, he fractured some ribs and tore the liver.

In the last moments of his fast-ebbing life, this sick, tired old man was not allowed to die in peace and dignity.

I encountered so many incidents similar to this one that I became preoccupied with the problem and finally felt compelled to write a book aimed at the medical profession on the subject of iatrogenic disease. In my introduction I made up a case that combined all the worst elements of several different cases of doctor-induced complications. Much to my horror, a year after the book's publication a real case was reported in the *Archives of Internal Medicine* duplicating my hypothetical nightmare almost exactly.

The fictitious case concerned a young man who had been

ill with the common cold. For this, his physician prescribed penicillin (absolutely useless for a virus infection). Ten days later, the patient reacted adversely to the penicillin with a troublesome rash covering his entire body. To alleviate the allergic reaction, the doctor now gave him a series of cortisone shots. As a consequence of the cortisone, an acute ulcer formed in his stomach and gave rise to a profuse hemorrhage. The patient was rushed to the hospital in a state of shock and over a period of five hours was given five transfusions. Three months went by; he recovered and was back on the job when a fellow worker remarked that his skin looked yellow. Alarmed, he hastened again to the doctor, who once more had him hospitalized. A series of tests led to a diagnosis of transfusion-incurred viral hepatitis. The damage to his liver from this blood-borne infection progressed to the cirrhotic (scarred) stage and he expired before the year was up.

I had written the book solely for the physician, in technical language that would exclude lay readers, on the theory that it would be harmful to tell the gory details of iatrogenesis to the public. After my book was released, this view was strengthened by an irresponsible article in a syndicated newspaper column that quoted from my book intemperately and out of context. When the column appeared, I was inundated with letters and phone calls from worried and anxious patients questioning the medications prescribed for them by their doctors. One man flew from Puerto Rico to New York to see me; he had stopped taking the medicine his doctor in San Juan had prescribed until he could consult me personally. The treatment prescribed by his physician had been clearly indicated and essential for his continued health; even a temporary interruption could have been harmful. He was one of many. I decided there were too many nervous people who would overreact to anything said on the subject, and in this way do themselves serious harm.

I believed the problem could be almost entirely corrected by physician education and peer review.

But a review of my book changed my mind: The reviewer for the *Annals of Internal Medicine* felt that my book would not achieve its intended objectives, because the very doctors who needed the lessons were the ones least likely to read it. This comment, the publication of a few well-written and constructive articles in the lay press, and the continued failure of physicians to react decisively and with more concern to this matter, changed my mind. I now believe continued patient and consumer education is essential if for no other reason than to stop the public from pressuring physicians to prescribe the latest miracle drugs. Exposure to facts can help the consumer realize that newness does not mean betterness and that a physician should not be judged according to the number of injections and the amount of medication he provides.

Allowing for the need to strengthen the drug licensing and testing procedures, the need to educate the consumer, and the need for closer supervision of the pharmaceutical industry, the crux of the matter must still be with the physician. He must take a leaf from that now almost extinct figure, the country doctor, and begin to look at his patients as total human beings with a past, a present, and a future. They are not merely an eye, a pain, or a kidney stone. Only then will he be able to apply the fruits of our scientific know-how with art, understanding, and compassion.

3. MYSTERY IN THE DARK—THE HEART-ATTACK TERROR

Look here we are being asked to respond to more terror than a civilized spirit can sustain. Considering the disagreeable terror glut, we must condition ourselves to discriminate amongst the sundry terrors to which we are daily exposed and to worry only about those few terrors which it is in our power to dispel or diminish.

Russell Baker, "The Terror Glut," New York *Times*

If 35 percent of his calories come from fats, is Junior being prepared starting in nursery school for a coronary occlusion? . . . Reviewing the dietaries of some of our teen-agers, I am struck by the resemblance to the diet that Olaf Michelsen uses to create obesity in rats. Frappes, fat-meat hamburgers, bacon-and-mayonnaise sandwiches, followed by ice cream, may be good for the farmer, good for the undertaker, and bad for the population. . . . Through the stimulation of advertising, tap water is being replaced by sugared juices and carbonated drinks. Snacks have become a ritualized part of the movies and are inseparably associated with television viewing.

Stanley Marion Garn, White House Conference on Children

Medicine is a science of uncertainty and an art of probability. . . . Absolute diagnoses are unsafe and are made at the expense of the conscience.

Sir William Osler

The more we learn about some things—such as heart attacks—the more complicated they become. The law defines fact differently from the way science does. The more engrossed I became in studying the enigmas of heart disease, the more aware I became of the schism between medical legalisms and medical science. Often, in medical research, anyone's guess is as good as an "educated" guess; from the same set of facts, one can come to two or more different logical conclusions. And yet, in many cases the law demands that medicine provide a definite answer. Some medical experts, whether for money or vanity, have allowed themselves to be caught up in this flattering search for the "oracular" answer, and in so doing have perverted truth.

Opinions that go beyond the limits of the accepted evidence may lead to miscarriages of justice, as happened—I believe—in a recent court case. The newspapers carried the story: A twenty-one-year-old man robbed a store run by a seventy-five-year-old woman. To keep her quiet, he tied her hands and feet. She died while he was robbing the cash register. In court, it was disclosed that she had had seriously advanced heart disease. The district attorney involved was trying to advance his career by piling up an impressive list of convictions and decided to go for a charge of murder, on the grounds that the victim had died as a direct result of the robber's actions. There was no sign of injury on the woman's body, and no one suggested that he had intended the woman any bodily harm.

The young man was found guilty of murder and sentenced to twenty-five years in jail after a highly respected medical examiner testified for the state that the woman had, without any doubt, died of "fright and exertion" after the thief had bound her.

There is little doubt that the woman died from heart failure. But is it fair to say that fright must have brought on the at-

254 POST-MORTEM

tack, beyond any reasonable doubt? There were cases under my jurisdiction as medical examiner in which psychological stress had to be given serious consideration as a likely precipitant of a lethal heart attack. An episode I vividly recall was the one of a father returning home from work who came upon the scene of his son in the act of stabbing his wife to death. Within minutes, he collapsed from a heart attack, and was dead within an hour. Was this mere coincidence, or was there a genuine cause-and-effect relationship between what he saw and his heart seizure? Such a thing is possible, but by no means is it the only possibility. And our system of justice demands that before a man can be convicted of murder, the case against him must be established beyond a reasonable doubt. It is frightening that the medical expert whose word directed the course of the trial had commented on a similar case on the opposite side some time before. In that case, a sixty-five-year-old delicatessan-store proprietor was held up; immediately after the robbery, the owner collapsed and died. The medical examiner said in an article on this case that the intangible and immeasurable nature of the emotional factors made them exceedingly difficult to evaluate. He said he couldn't deny the possibility that the robbery and the heart attack were coincidental. In the latter case, the medical examiner had no vested interest; the article was an intellectual exercise. In the first case, he was pledged to uphold the interests of the state—and unfortunately he included among these interests the importance of racking up murder convictions. And he was not without self-interest: It was certainly a lack of humility that urged him to testify so positively about an issue on which there is much scientific debate. According to legal authorities, only one similar conviction has been found in the local legal archives, and that was nearly a century ago.

It is disconcerting when the same set of facts can serve one interest one day and serve another the next—especially when a young man's future is at stake.

Of course, vested interests aren't always vicious. There are times when the most conscientious and honest researcher can have an unconscious bias in favor of his own preconceived ideas. It happened to me when I was doing studies on heart disease. I was trying to correlate body type with increased tendencies toward heart attack. What I did was to study one hundred hearts and measure the size of the arteriosclerotic formations encroaching on the main arterial channels (which feed blood to the heart muscle). I then related this to the observed physical characteristics (age, sex, bodily features) of the deceased individual to whom the heart had belonged. To my satisfaction, my original hypothesis was substantiated.

When I discussed the results with colleagues in the same field, they cast doubt on my absolutely definitive findings. They discreetly advised me to repeat the measurements on the coronary arteries, and suggested that this time I should use the "double blind" method to forestall any extraneous subjective influences from creeping into the measurements. The first time around, I had tagged the hearts and stored them in containers of formaldehyde. For the repeat study, I ordered the laboratory assistant to relabel all the specimens with a secret code known only to him. The code was not to be broken until all measurements had been completed. Now, without any hint as to the specific source of each heart, I was automatically precluded from relating the new measurements, as they were being made, to the specific characteristics of any particular individual. The sum of the findings on this second attempt still supported my views but not as decisively as before.

I realized after this new set of measurements that, without any overt awareness on my part, I must have stretched or perhaps shrunk a measurement here and there to make them fit more neatly into the pattern of my projected hypothesis. Right now, I still believe I was not intentionally dishonest, at least not on a conscious level. Experienced and authoritative scientists with unquestioned integrity long ago recognized that this behavior is within the nature of the beast and developed the "double-blind" method, which is now accepted routine, especially when testing the safety and efficacy of newly formulated drugs. The evaluator of the medication is purposely kept in the dark and does not know which of the patients in the study group are receiving the genuine and active drug and which are getting an inert imitation. At the other end of the double-blind study, the patients are uninformed as to whether they are being treated with the active medicine or with an inactive simulation of the real pill. Hopefully, this procedure tends to reinforce the investigator's objectivity in gathering the facts, and limits the patients' subjective responses to the anticipated effects of the treatment. Surprisingly, even these precautions are not entirely foolproof.

On a wider scale, one can take all the facts into account and still come up with an incomplete theory if all the logically possible explanations aren't weighed at the same time. For example, I had been puzzling over the reasons why two individuals with identical amounts of disease blocking the flow of blood to their heart muscles had different outcomes when stricken with heart attacks. One could die almost instantaneously, and the other might suffer slight damage to his heart and then recover to resume normal life activities.

Heart-disease experts have known that when a coronary artery is closed off, nature responds by providing blood vessels that can detour the flow of blood past this obstruction. It occurred to me that perhaps the ones who die instantly have failed to develop enough of these bypasses to sustain life in the presence of a heart attack, while the survivors have developed a good supply of these auxiliary channels. The question then was how to go about proving this.

I was at an impasse until one day I came across a technique developed by another investigator designed to show the presence of these bypasses when examining the hearts at autopsy. It consisted of injecting small glass beads suspended in fluid into the arterial channel above the obstruction and checking to see if these pellets came out on the side past the obstruction. If so, it meant the pellets had passed around the block by a detour. Using this method, I studied the hearts of men who had died suddenly from heart attacks and compared them with hearts from men who had survived the heart attack only to die at a later date for other reasons.

Detours were found only in a rare few of the sudden fatalities but were always present in the survivors. This seemed to confirm my original views, and I reported this conclusion in an article in a prominent medical journal. One day, in a discussion of this matter with a colleague, he insisted I had not proved my concept to the exclusion of other theories. He suggested that these detours could just as well have developed *because* the patient survived, and were not necessarily the reason for the survival. He was absolutely right. His conclusion was just as valid as mine. I had proved nothing.

Unlike the medical examiner in the court case I've just described, I'm inclined to hedge my bets when I'm called as an expert. A case I'll call the Dowd case provides a perfect example of the need for flexibility and the imperfect state of our knowledge about heart disease.

I was called to testify at a workmen's-compensation hearing concerning a possible work-related heart-attack fatality. I had conducted the autopsy on the body of the deceased. Mr. Dowd was fifty-six. He had been employed for twenty-six years as a public school custodian in central Westchester. On the eventful day, he was trimming the lawn with a power mower. The task was a moderate one and the physical effort required was minimal: the energy expended was well within his usual daily range. George Watkins, his helper, was close behind, gathering up the cuttings. They had been at this job for no more than thirty minutes when Watkins heard Dowd groan. He looked over and saw his boss clutching and rubbing his chest with both hands as if in severe pain. Immediately, Dowd fell to the ground, and in the process struck the back of his head on the ground. Though still visibly breathing, he was motionless. Watkins ran for the school nurse. When she arrived, Dowd seemed lifeless, but because the nurse felt a pulse beating feebly, she started mouth-to-mouth respiration and kept at it until the ambulance arrived fifteen minutes later. The ambulance technicians attempted external cardiac massage and applied mechanical resuscitation—all to no avail. The heart never started up again. Upon arrival of the doctor, all that remained was to pronounce the heart-attack victim dead.

The moment our mortuary ambulance left to pick up the remains of Mr. Dowd, my staff, trained in the processing of sudden deaths, began to seek out all the background information the department would need for an eventual medicolegal ruling. I had prepared a special questionnaire for this purpose; and I had also added questions designed to aid my research study, which was concerned with pinpointing the environmental culprits responsible for striking down at least fifteen adults in the United States from "heart attacks" each day. Dowd's helper, Mr. Watkins, supplied us with the important details of the final episode. He described his boss's behavior and activities in the two hours preceding his death. He stated that, until the last few minutes, he had noticed nothing untoward.

For years I have felt that careful study of the period close to the time of the heart attack will uncover critical secrets that will lead to a more rational understanding of this problem. But this endeavor is partially frustrated by the fact that many of these fatalities go unwitnessed, leaving no one to supply the vital information. Furthermore some investigators have unthinkingly lumped together the witnessed and unwitnessed cases and have formed conclusions that have produced a distorted picture of what really occurs in the final moments of these sudden heart-attack fatalities.

George Watkins told me the attack had come on suddenly, "like a bolt of lightning," and that it was all over within minutes. There was no time, under the best of conditions, to secure the kind of medical aid able to check the fast-moving lethal chain of events. When Mrs. Dowd arrived at our offices to identify her husband's body, she told me that Mr. Dowd had appeared in good health and had no reason for visiting his physician in the previous three years. As far as she knew, he didn't have heart disease. His blood pressure, taken by an insurance-company doctor, was normal as recently as two months before his death. He was a heavy cigarette smoker. One key piece of information was revealed while I was carefully probing into the last two weeks of her husband's life. This was the fact that he had complained of "heartburn and indigestion" one week previously. This lasted two days, but he was not incapacitated and went to work.

Although Dowd had not been examined by his personal physician for several years, I still contacted him. He confirmed what we already had learned from the widow. The school authorities also gave their former custodian a clean bill of health, in the form of an excellent work-attendance record. I also learned that his duties never required more than moderate exertion.

For the purposes of my research project, I had set up a work-activity classification based on levels of energy expenditure.

Those jobs with the least output of physical work were labeled sedentary and were represented by clerks, accountants, bank tellers, office managers, and business executives. Next in order came those with moderate activity, represented by letter carriers, waiters, house painters, and delivery men. Then came strenuous activity, represented by truck loaders, steam fitters, and road workers. Dowd fitted into the moderate category.

Review of the information gathered at the time of the autopsy revealed two relevant items. The first was the complaint of "heartburn and indigestion" a few days prior to death, which may have been an earlier indication of the beginnings of Dowd's heart attack. In this case, the attack could have been in progress days before he was pushing the power lawn mower. The second was the fact that Dowd was a heavy cigarette smoker. The cigarette habit, at least statistically, is more closely associated with sudden fatal coronary deaths than is unusual physical stress. My recent studies in this area point to an extension of the sudden-heart-attack epidemic to women, who until recently were relatively immune. This change appears related to the increase in heavy smoking in women.

More knowledge of Dowd's life style and personal habits might have been helpful, but he was the only one who could have supplied it. Promptness in digging out all the essential facts guarantees a fairly accurate and complete story. As the interval increases from the point of death to the time of interrogation, the answers tend to become less informative and reliable. This emphasizes the urgency of early interviews. Otherwise the participants—the widow, the helper, the employer, and the family physician—develop second thoughts and can mull over the affair as it affects their personal stake in the final outcome. A lengthy interval permits lawyers or friends to advise, caution, or even coach those concerned on how much and what to reveal. The longer the lapse, the hazier becomes one's memory for the pertinent details. Given the time to think, the school employers worry about being accused of negligence in maintaining unsafe working conditions. The size of their insurance premiums is dependent on the amount and number of compensation awards to their employees. Mr. Watkins, the helper, could color his story one way if he was friendly with Dowd's family or another way to curry favor with the school authorities. The widow, on advice of counsel, could have conveniently neglected to recall the "heartburn" episode. The family doctor might desire to cover up an oversight in his last examination of Dowd. These modifications, appearing superficially inconsequential, could be decisive in swinging a judgment in either direction. And as for the needs of my research, the distortions or outright falsifications could render conclusions, painstakingly arrived at after years of collecting data, completely invalid. Conscious of all these pitfalls, I insisted on learning all I could about each case the moment a death notification was received.

As usual, before making the initial incision into Mr. Dowd's body I searched for any external changes that might bear on a logical interpretation of the sequence of events leading to the fatality. Mr. Watkins had previously told us about Dowd's head striking the ground. A small and superficial bruise was noted on the scalp at the site of the impact. The turf where he fell was soft and the injury was only skin deep, with no skull or brain damage. I dismissed the bruise as having no influence on the course of events. In other cases, extensive head injuries produced under similar circumstances have confused the issue. If the head injury is minor, the victim could conceivably survive the heart attack; or else the head injury in and of itself can be lethal. In the latter instance the evidence of underlying or pre-existing heart disease is entirely coincidental and non-contributory to the death. In some situations—for example, a car wreck—the autopsy reveals a skull fracture, brain injuries, and diseased coronary arteries. Independent of each other, the head damage or the heart disease can kill fast. The medical examiner is expected to come up with a plausible explanation of the event. He asks himself certain questions in an attempt to reconstruct the sequence of events. Did the driver lose control of the car because of a heart seizure? Was a mechanical defect in the car or road the primary cause of the smashup? If the accident came first, did it bring on the heart attack? Was the death entirely due to the brain damage from the impact against the windshield? All are distinct possibilities.

Usually it is necessary to go beyond the autopsy to find the answer. At that, one may never be certain. And yet, unhesitatingly, positive opinions are invariably sworn to under oath in court. I was subpoenaed by the compensation bureau to present the facts of the post-mortem examination on Dowd. In the course of my testimony, the nature of the questions changed from ones requiring factual responses to ones necessitating opinions. The referee, aware of this, temporarily halted the proceedings to alter my status as a witness from one who was called upon only for facts to one who was qualified as an expert in the medical specialty bearing on this case. I could therefore present authoritative opinions. This meant I was now required to answer questions on the mechanisms and causes of heart attacks.

The court wanted to know my views on the connection, if any, between Mr. Dowd's physical efforts while working and the precipitation of his fatal heart attack. The defense attorney representing the insurance fund wanted to disprove any causal relationship between the job and the fatality, so as to prevent a ruling that would award financial compensation to Dowd's widow. He introduced his first question with a preliminary display and quote from a publication describing a

study of mine on the association of different levels of occupational physical activity and exertion with the frequency of
sudden fatal heart attacks. This investigation was based on all
the sudden-death cases in Westchester County autopsied during
my tenure as medical examiner. At the time, it was the most
comprehensive report on the subject in the medical literature.
The lawyer had done his homework well in discovering and
reading this article, and with this information hoped to box
me in with an answer favoring his cause.

He asked: "Isn't it true, in this study of yours you have presented convincing evidence to prove there is in all likelihood
little or no causal connection between strenuous physical activity at work and the precipitation of sudden death from arteriosclerotic heart disease, and in those few occasions where
excessive hard work has been performed immediately prior to
an unexpected death from this disease, the number of such
events has been uncommon, forcing you to conclude that in
most cases it was probably a statistical coincidence, bearing
no direct influence on the ultimate catastrophe?"

To this lengthy, and cleverly worded, question I had no
choice but to answer "Yes—those were my conclusions,
but . . ."

No sooner had I said this, and even before there was a chance
to qualify my seemingly categorical response, than the opposing
attorney confronted me with the other critical question. This
interruption by plaintiff's attorney was permitted because compensation trials are conducted in a somewhat informal manner.
Testimony is taken under oath and the adversary system is
practiced, but the usual trial procedure of completing the direct
examination before cross-examination is not routinely followed.
Nor are the rules of evidence as rigid.

The question from Mrs. Dowd's lawyer was: "But, Dr. Spain,
isn't it equally a fact that in your duties as a medical examiner

you were sometimes required to investigate and also autopsy
the bodies of men suddenly stricken dead while shoveling snow?
And in this connection, isn't it also a fact that these 'heart-
attack' deaths occurring during episodes of severe exertion
add to the number of sudden fatalities seen by you during the
winter months?"

Again, and without the slightest hesitation, I answered,
"Yes." Here, too, I had planned to offer some qualifying remarks, but I didn't get a chance. The juxtaposed affirmative answer coming in rapid succession to seemingly antagonistic
questions brought forth an incredulous expression on her hon-
or's face. "I've never heard the likes of this. Aren't you speaking out of both sides of your mouth at the same time?"

"Your honor," I replied, "I realize my statements were contradictory but I regret I am unable to be more definitive. This
is the current state of knowledge, or perhaps, more realistically,
the lack of knowledge in this perplexing area of heart disease."
I was most respectful to the court when saying this, but I failed
to soothe the ruffled feelings of the referee. She curtly dismissed
me from the witness stand. "There will be no further need for
your opinions. You are discharged from the proceedings."

Her attitude in this case, and that of the attorneys, the insurance companies, the expert medical witnesses, and the vast
bureaucratic apparatus handling the compensation matter was
not atypical. All viewed this medical problem, still unsolved
two decades after that trial, in an oversimplified way. The referee, beset by the endless calendar of protracted and unfinished
cases, had one aim: to get the case over with once and for all.
For this she needed someone to give her an authoritative and
conclusive opinion. She didn't care which side it favored, only
that she could use it to end the case. The attorney for the state
insurance fund, as a representative of a public agency theo-
retically neutral, had an inordinate interest in his own career, in

this case best served by saving money for the insurance fund. His presentation was as biased as the plaintiff's attorney, whose fee was directly proportional to the size of the award. The well-paid, suave medical experts, with equal assurance, offered absolute diagnoses on either side of the case. Their courtroom demeanor and their dogmatism never finds its counterpart when they render opinions on their own patients in the privacy of their offices.

Actually the doctors, lawyers, referees, and all others making up the casts of these compensation cases should not be faulted for a socioeconomic system that avoids direct responsibility for the fate of the hapless survivors. Compassionate and understanding witnesses frequently do look the other way and stretch medical reason to provide for these destitute people. Unfortunately, subterfuge has been substituted as the mechanism for handling a human problem that should be openly and honestly solved by the community as a whole. I was pleased that my hasty dismissal from the hearing did not prejudice the widow's chances for an equitable settlement from the school's insurers, because the essential findings of the autopsy performed by me two years back had already been incorporated into the trial record. I was pleased that the final verdict favored Mrs. Dowd.

The referee's failure to comprehend the innuendos and limitations inherent in my answers prompted her to accuse me of double talk. Had I been permitted to expand my remarks, she might not have been so perplexed. A clear distinction would have been made between two processes: the chronic underlying disease, arteriosclerosis, and the acute event, the sudden heart attack. Arteriosclerosis develops slowly and insidiously over many years and has its own set of causes, some known and others still undiscovered. The second—the precipitous fatality coming on in minutes—has a different set of causes. Habitually

sustained physical activity appears to slow down the advance
of the arteriosclerotic disease, while, in the acute event, unusual
physical strain may be harmful. Given the opportunity to explain this to the court might have clarified matters.

It was precisely at this point, where my interests veered from
the legal to the purely medical aspects of arteriosclerosis, that
I faced up to the perverted uses of suggestive but still unproved
theories. Though here and there I had been familiar with an
occasional scientist who for opportunistic gain committed
crimes against the pursuit of truth, I had not been exposed in
this field of research to the same blatant distortions experienced
in the cigarette-smoking controversy. But I soon found there
were many trying to make material gain from the knowledge
about heart attacks that was slowly beginning to emerge from
the scientific assembly line.

The dairy industry, for example, played both ends against
the middle. While their public-relations men daily extolled the
virtues of whole milk for the growth and development of
the child, they at the same time catered to the new demands
of an increasingly heart-disease-conscious group of consumers
who were looking for foods with less saturated fats and cholesterol. The industry met this challenge by repackaging and re-
labeling the old-time unpopular skim milk with more attractive
wrappings and names and then charging more for it than they
charged for whole milk. For years the dairy lobby succeeded
in preventing the supposedly safer vegetable oils, in the form
of oleomargarine, from having a fair competitive place in the
market. Earlier in the game, they subsidized those researchers
who opposed the high fat-cholesterol factor as an important
cause for the increase in heart attacks and sponsored even
more generously those scientists who placed the main blame
elsewhere.

The fish industry seized the moment to capitalize on scien-

tists' pronouncements that meat products were high in cholesterol to promote such slogans as "Eat fish daily and live longer"
and "Fish foods prevent heart attacks." Clearly these are not
medically proven facts. The corn-oil-products industry took advantage of the medical momentum seemingly in their favor by
promoting the less-saturated vegetable oils with a cleverly
worded and highly health-oriented advertising campaign. In
pushing the sale of corn-oil oleomargarine, they neglected to
stress the fact that they partially saturate it to make it more
palatable. At many of the national heart-disease conventions
they selectively invited to lavish cocktail parties those scientists whose work favored their cause. Ironically they served
quantities of shrimp fried in corn oil at these affairs. Shrimp are
loaded with cholesterol.

The drug industry put its best chemists to work to develop
drugs capable of eliminating or lessening the amount of cholesterol in the blood. These compounds were rushed to the market,
and the pharmaceutical houses directed a saturation advertising
attack on physicians, pushing the great attributes of these medicaments. No one has as yet demonstrated that the lowering of
cholesterol in the blood, artificially by the use of medicine, can
slow down the progression of arteriosclerosis. Despite this, the
sales of these drugs brought drug companies millions of dollars.
Some of these drugs caused considerable harm and had to be
withdrawn from use. The others remain of doubtful value.
Sadly, many doctors, in their ignorance about the true nature
of this disease, were willing partners in this commercial venture.

Because of a lack of rational national, over-all planning,
financing of individual research has been at best precarious
and sometimes disheartening. I have seen men sell their souls
for adequate money sorely needed for essential projects. Fortunately my early studies required little funding and were carried out at an initial cost of seventy-five dollars, used to buy

a small pump for injecting the coronary arteries. As the work progressed, the problems increased, and the need for a more sophisticated and multivaried approach became increasingly apparent. The costs rose proportionately. Over the course of the next ten years, I spent approximately a quarter of a million dollars on the investigations growing out of the original work. This seems like a huge sum, but by today's standards it is a drop in the bucket. The funds were obtained from diverse sources: among them, governmental agencies, private foundations, and generous individuals. The sum of money allotted in the earlier days of arteriosclerosis investigation was a shabby pittance compared to the funds poured into the study of other, less significant diseases; close working contact on several levels with the public and private national research effort disclosed to me a succession of harsh conflicts over money. Every segment of the research area was partially tarnished and hindered by these anti-social displays. Fortunately, then and as always, there existed alongside this ugly scene a large group of devoted doctors and scientists whose interest was the common good. For the others, the smaller group, the welfare of the public never entered determinations of where the money should be spent. Those with the powerful political connections, with the slickest public-relations departments, and with the least respect for the truth they were seeking, too often received the lion's share of available research grants. The funds were given without regard for legitimate priorities of health needs.

Heart attacks were incorrectly regarded as limited to the elderly, and so received short shrift because of our false standards concerning the aged: that they no longer actively contribute to the growth of our gross national product. Arteriosclerosis was a relatively orphaned affliction.

In contrast, infantile-paralysis research was a success from the beginning. "Polio," still in the historical period of its viru-

lent epidemics, occupied the public's chief attention. The horror
of witnessing innocent children, playful and full of life one day
and dead the next day or else crippled for life, filled everyone
with fear, anxiety, and compassion. The nation was mobilized
to conquer this scourge. The national polio foundation and
lesser groups concerned with this disease had merely to nod and
the money poured in. The plethora of contributions created a
surplus that could have been rationally spread out. Yet a sense
of similarity of interest and co-operation was lacking to a degree
that precluded the overly rich polio groups from channeling
some of the excess into other, needy research areas. Irrational
sentimentality and excessive organizational self-interest ran
roughshod over socially oriented requirements.

Slowly the climate for heart research began to change. In
1956 I received an invitation to participate in the first Arden
House Conference on Coronary Heart Disease and High Blood
Pressure. This meeting was organized by the National Heart
Institute and the American Heart Association. It brought together for the first time, for a week of intensive workshop sessions, twenty doctors and scientists of varied disciplines who
were concerned with mounting a mass research effort to com-
bat the heart-attack problem. At the conclusion of this conference, the group issued a report spelling out where we were
and where we had to go to resolve this problem. It was sent
to all institutions and scientists concerned with arteriosclerosis
and served as a stimulus for many of the important and long-
range studies that were carried out in the next decade. Almost
overnight, arteriosclerosis research received top priority from
the granting agencies. The realities of this devastating disease
had finally created a more favorable climate for work in this
area. However, I am convinced that the speed with which the
attitude toward research in this area changed was due to something revealed to us by Dr. Ray Trussel in his opening remarks

as chairman of the Arden House meeting. In tracing the origins of this conference, he pointed out that Dwight Eisenhower (at that time President), Lyndon Johnson, and a number of leading congressmen had recently suffered heart attacks. In other words, a vested interest intruded: the legislators' personal involvement with this disease produced immediate results. A Congressional committee held a hearing on the subject, and the Surgeon General was charged with mounting a massive urgent effort to solve the problem of coronary-artery disease. In addition, Dr. Paul Dudley White, the most eminent cardiologist in the country, had been summoned in consultation on President Eisenhower's case. Dr. White for years had been the leading proponent of expanding heart-disease research. I am sure this also helped the cause.

With money available, the race was on to get there first. Institutions openly competed with each other, as in the business world, for a scarce and essential commodity—in this case, the competent technicians and scientists. Soon they were all gobbled up: Epidemiologists, biochemists, statisticians, research-oriented clinicians, and experimentalists were in short supply. The highest bidders and the most prestigious institutions grabbed the most and the best. Rival groups stole scientists from each other to improve their grant-seeking posture. Co-operative endeavor was not the order of the day. The money, the time, the brains could have been more gainfully employed and could have shortened the time spent in seeking the crucial answers needed to save lives. We have lived too long within the aura of the entrepreneurs' individualistic, fiercely competitive, dog-eat-dog business world's value system. Some of it couldn't help rubbing off on the scientific community.

I vividly recall the sharp debates in the councils of the American Heart Association over attempts to launch co-operative ventures among different research groups. Among the farsighted were Dr. Jeremiah Stamler, noted for his many contributions in the prevention of coronary heart disease; Dr. Felix Moore, a leading biostatistician for the National Heart Institute; and Dr. Frederick Epstein, the clinical epidemiologist who headed up the committee eventually formed to augment co-operative studies. At first the going was rough. Only a few combined efforts got off the ground. Now these are commonplace. An early successful enterprise resulted from the Public Health Service-sponsored Framingham study joining forces with the Albany heart-study group. From this effort emerged the most definitive proof of the deleterious effect of cigarette smoking on the heart.

Those who worked for co-operative endeavors were acutely cognizant of the reasons for the past failure of joint undertakings. There were many difficulties in reconciling the organizational, technical, and research differences among the various groups. Whose project design was to be accepted? What about the control and distribution of the funds? How was credit for discoveries to be apportioned? Who was to have the honor of making the first presentation of the findings at the scientific-association meetings? Most of these obstacles had in the past nullified the successful implementation of combined efforts. The issue was ultimately forced by necessity. The studies required to finally nail down the answers on diet were of such magnitude—demanding such vast outlays of money, so many pressures, and so much time, in order to study populations of more than fifty thousand people—that no one group could dream of going it alone. Good sense and common goals dictated what had to be done.

Before the national Diet and Coronary Heart Disease Study was to finally become a reality, yet another obstacle had to be overcome. For a long time, a fundamental difference has existed in the approach toward disease between public-health-oriented

physicians and the doctors who tend to the immediate daily
needs of patients. The former are oriented toward prevention
of disease and the latter toward the repair or alleviation of illness already present. With a chronic disease, such as arteriosclerosis, which extends for decades in the lifetime of one
individual, the two come out fighting on the allocation of funds
essential to carrying out the long-range investigation to determine the best preventative measures. The clinically trained,
practicing physicians were preoccupied with their daily overwhelming problem of helping people survive in the face of advanced and irreparable damage to their hearts. The public-health
approach, taking the long view, was expending every effort to
prevent this damage from occurring in the first place. The way
the money would be spent depended on the views of those in
control of the purse strings. There should have been room for
both, but there wasn't. For a while, control was dominated by
the terminal patchwork, repair approach—favoring doctors who
could produce for the public concrete, visible results. This path,
though resulting in short-lived effects, with its heart transplants,
mechanical hearts, and glamorized surgical procedures, caught
the popular fancy. The important dietary study was delayed,
because the funds were diverted to headline-catching activities.
It took time, and the failure of their short-term methods, before
good sense finally prevailed. The one meaningful investigation,
capable of producing the information needed to add years of
healthy and useful life to individuals who would otherwise die
in their prime, has finally been launched by the Heart and Lung
Institute of HEW.

It began as a massive, national dietary study, but has since
been emasculated. Even though its original size and design have
been compromised, I still feel that within the next five years
it will yield sufficient information to convince the medical profession and the public of the harmful role of excessive animal

fats and cholesterol in the causation of coronary heart disease. With this proof we can then anticipate the inevitable fight to unseat the bull, the cow, and their creamy by-products from the throne of the food kingdom in order to put in their formerly eminent place the fish and the stringbean. Imagine the intensity of the battle to do away with the Madison Avenue court jesters and install in their place informed and responsible nutritionists as health advisers. Having previously been scarred and personally humiliated in the struggle of cigarette smoking versus cancer, I can testify that the dairy and beef trusts along with the hamburger and custard stands will not willingly or gracefully relinquish one penny of their highly remunerative interests.

But, long before the present research stage was reached, there was for a period a shortage of well-trained technicians and scientific workers in the bioscience fields. This is hard to believe in view of the present-day unemployment plight of Ph.D.s, but the shortage existed and it hampered the coronary-research effort. Nothing much was being done about this scarce commodity until, one morning, the nation woke up to the news of the successful Russian launching of Sputnik 1. This stirred the Washington manpower experts into action, now alarmed by what they considered a serious threat to the nation's vital interests. They rapidly prepared a program for expanding our scientific and technical reserves. Their prime concern was with the development of aerospace and military hardware, but other areas of science benefited from the rub-off.

In this process, I became involved in an unexpected undertaking, one closely tied to the heart-attack problem. The nation was still gripped by the cold-war hysteria. When the short-lived excitement and admiration for the Soviet achievement subsided, it was replaced by a sobering thought: the Russians are ahead of us. Responding to this, the Squibb Foundation contributed a generous sum of money to the American Heart Association to be utilized for an educational campaign designed to encourage more of the nation's youth to enter scientific pursuits. To implement this plan, the heart association produced ten films to be televised nationally and to be shown throughout the country's schools. Each production highlighted a special aspect of research into heart disease and featured one investigator and his research project. My project was selected for one of these half-hour shows, probably because it lent itself to a dramatic visual presentation and because it showed the need for more epidemiologists, biochemists, doctors, statisticians, bioengineers, nutritionists, computer technologists, etc.

The series was called "Decision for Research" and the film I was featured in was entitled *Mystery in the Dark*. My show traced my investigations into some of the possible causes of heart attacks: diet, lack of exercise, cigarette smoking, high blood pressure, and inherited constitutional vulnerability. In the course of the presentation, I discussed the varied motivations for going into research and the deep personal sense of fulfillment from these endeavors. First the productions were televised live over the National Educational TV network, and at a later date they were presented over the NBC network. The public's reception was highly favorable, and the heart association began scheduling showings throughout the country. Unfortunately, before the films were ever released for the first school showings, a major national scandal hit a key figure of the cast, and the entire series of films was buried in the association's inactive files. Charles Van Doren, hired at the suggestion of a public-relations consultant, was the moderator of each show. Van Doren, a youthful, handsome, and debonair professor of English literature at Columbia University, had achieved national fame and fortune by answering correctly the $64,000 Question on the popular television quiz show. A new type of youth hero had appeared on the scene, one admired for his intellect. So, to add a bit of dash to the series, he was retained by the producers and subsequently appeared in each film.

But disaster struck, and Charles Van Doren's bubble burst. Along with others, Van Doren was charged with having participated in the advance rigging of quiz shows. The conspirators were accused of having fixed the questions and answers before ever appearing in public. The heart association's project, the months of planning, the efforts of the scientists, and the expectation of reaching the minds of young people and inspiring them in the pursuit of truth all went down the drain. Charles Van Doren, the magnet selected to attract a youthful audience, had been allegedly exposed as a fraud, destroyed by his selfish, short-sighted opportunism.

Despite so much tawdry behavior, the mean and petty diversions, and the many masquerading faces of self-interest, the basic core of the research world single-mindedly continues to fit into their proper places the numerous irregular parts of this complicated, scientific puzzle. Progress is still made.

It is heartening to me, for example, that the unprecedented co-operative dietary study will soon produce the essential tools for reversing the ravages of arteriosclerotic heart disease. The next unavoidable step will be to alter our culturally and geo-economically determined overindulgent, deeply ingrained, and admittedly pleasurable eating habits. Major changes will be required. The ubiquitous television athlete, whose maximum daily physical exercise comes when he reluctantly tears himself away from the viewing box during the commercial interlude to grab a cream-rich snack from the deep freeze, will have to mend his ways. This is, as I see it, the only way out of this modern terror.

I personally felt twenty years ago that enough evidence had been accumulated to indicate that excessive amounts of animal fats and cholesterol were a significant factor in the increase of heart attacks in younger males. Females are protected by the estrogen hormone prior to menopause, so don't have to worry about cholesterol. Women who smoke do have to worry about heart attacks, as cigarettes wipe out the natural advantage of the estrogen. I made certain changes in my eating habits twenty years ago. I love to eat, and I like all kinds of food, but I began by giving up whole milk, butter, cream-rich and shortening-saturated desserts such as Danish pastry, and fatty meats soaked in gravy. I drank coffee black, switched to the leaner cuts of meat, and ate more fish. Eggs were eliminated. Sausage and bacon are also poor choices for breakfast foods. On occasion I break my rules: I never insult a hostess when I have been invited for dinner by refusing the fancy dessert she has labored over, but I limit the size of my portion. There are times, when I am traveling or on vacation, when it is impossible to resist eating one of those big, old-fashioned breakfasts. My main weakness is cheese, but I have always avoided the processed ones, to which butter fat has been added. I enjoy eating fresh fruits and vegetables both for their taste (which is a refreshing change in this day of artificially sweetened, prepackaged con-venience foods) and for their nutritive value. I have never smoked cigarettes.

I have always been physically active and for many years have played tennis all year round, on the average of twice a week. Lately I have added swimming several times each week to my activities. This is not looked upon as medical treatment. I enjoy it.

How many years of health this has or will add to my life I have no way of knowing; but in the light of my work, and exposure daily to deaths from heart attacks, I feel the better for it. I recommend these modifications to all my friends, but no one should ever make drastic changes in his living habits without the supervision of his physician.

Incidentally I am a firm believer in stress as an inevitable, unalterable, and even essential part of life. I have never been disturbed by it or tried to avoid it.

There is a widely held impression that top business executives, under constant tension, are more prone to heart attacks than their underlings and the menial workers. It probably will surprise most who believe this that all the studies done under the most rigidly controlled methods have failed to support this view. Du Pont's study on its employees was noteworthy in that, over a three-year period, initial heart attacks after the age of forty-five occurred more frequently among lower-salaried male employees than those in the higher brackets. Men in the highest pay bracket had the lowest rate of heart attacks. The study also concluded that responsibilities attached to a job are not an indicator of how much stress a man undergoes. Other investigations tend to confirm the findings of the Du Pont study. Most feel that the amount of, or rather the lack of, physical activity on or off the job may be a more important consideration. Formerly, blue-collar workers received more exercise on their jobs than executives. But now, with automation, it's reversing: blue-collar workers get little exercise on the job and less when they go home and turn on the television set; executives often play squash twice a week, year round. Typical of leading cardiologists' attitudes on the question of stress is that of Dr. E. Grey Dimond of the University of Missouri Medical School, who says, "I work and drive as hard as I am capable and fully believe that I would have found or made life just as stressful had I lived in ancient Egypt, in Greece, or in Rome. . . . I do not personally feel stressed and do not believe modern living, or my version of it, has changed my survival time one day."

The "broken" heart, the "quickened" pulse, and the "pounding" heartbeat have been the classic symbols novelists and poets use to denote such emotions as fear, anxiety, guilt, despair, and unrequited love. But these same irregularities of the heartbeat are equally symptomatic of positive and highly pleasurable or rewarding feelings, such as fulfilled love and excited, joyful anticipation. To me it appears that the available evidence in support of the emotional causation of heart attacks has not yet earned an enduring place among our serious scientific concepts, and for the moment would better be consigned to our literature of folklore and tales of romance. The day may come when convincing proof exists, but it is not yet at hand.

EPILOGUE: OUR THROWAWAY SOCIETY

The death of any man diminishes me for I am involved in mankind. . . .

John Donne, Devotions XVII

After seeing so many violent and unnecessary deaths, I have come to feel, perhaps more so than most people, that in recent years there has been a relentless succession of violations of the human spirit. We see more and more brutalization: murder, sniping, rape, hijacking, kidnaping, mugging—and seem to respond less and less to it. When a more-harrowing-than-usual event occurs, pointing up the lesser horrors we ignore, we refuse to believe it. Something like that happened at Attica during the prison rebellion. I was involved only peripherally on a professional level, but what I saw and heard was enough to make me realize that no one wants to believe how dehumanized humanity has become.

I think the general public responded with shock and sorrow to the waste at Attica of human life—of the lives of the dead guards and prisoners both. But what it could not accept, and as a result refused to believe, was that the guards had not been mutilated and killed by the rebelling prisoners, but were shot

by the attacking troops—their own side. Dr. John Edland, the
Monroe County medical examiner, respected as a reputable
forensic pathologist by the community, became overnight a target for professional attack when he disclosed that the guards
had been shot by their own men. His autopsies on the eight
guards' bodies failed to reveal any slashed throats or mutilated
bodies. They had been killed by bullets.

Coming as it did right after the prison officials' version of
the rebellion—that the hostages were being tortured and an attack was launched to save them—Dr. Edland's autopsy report
caused an unpleasant stir. Two forensic pathologists from other
parts of the state were hastily summoned to the scene to re-
examine the bodies. Their findings did not differ from his.
Nevertheless, the attempts to have Dr. Edland give testimony
about his report before any of the investigative bodies dealing
with Attica were frustrated. He spoke out publicly on the entire
affair at the annual national session of the American Academy
of Forensic Sciences. From the podium, he openly discussed
the official neglect of his reports and said, in effect, that he
felt like a public official without a public constituency. This boy-
cott of a respected public official was the obverse of the all-
too-eager belief in the earlier statements of the prison officials,
depicting hostages with slashed throats, broken arms, broken
faces, and other gory details of mutilation. On September 15,
1971, the New York *Times* reported how the local townspeople
responded to Dr. Edland's findings: "The reaction of disbelief
was widespread and strongly felt in the all-white town, whose
main industry is a maximum-security prison with a population
of inmates 85% non-white or Spanish speaking."

What is it about Attica that people can't face? It isn't what
the rebellion says about the quality of life in our prisons that
the public rejects. The public has been told about it by many,
including former Attorney General John Mitchell, who is not

usually regarded as a staunch champion of human rights: "The state of America's prisons comes close to a national shame. No civilized society should allow it to continue." Mitchell is quoted by Ben Bagdikian in his book *The Shame of the Prisons*. Bagdikian concludes: "Human prisoners in the United States are more carelessly handled than animals in the zoo, which have more space and get more care."

This kind of realization fails to explain the deep moral anguish about Attica that persisted more than a year later. Everyone wants to bury it, to deny it, to rearrange the memories as if it were only a bad dream. People are frightened at what a hard look might uncover.

What was the reasoning behind the hasty decision for the massive armed assault? From the very onset, there was an irrevocable determination not to compromise on amnesty; to cut off all negotiations at the right moment; and to launch a scorching and unsparing intervention. It is now clear that no alternative course ever received serious thought, the lives of the hostages notwithstanding.

Given the antiquated attitudes and past practices of those in charge, it could not have been otherwise. After all, one does not trifle with authority; one does not make deals with hardened criminals, with outcasts. Once and for all, said the prison officials, the line must be drawn and an example set; a sign of weakness could stimulate a flurry of prison outbreaks across the nation. We have a sacred duty to the rest of the country. These stagnant views were fertile soil for any suggestion that some of the guards had already been mutilated; the suggestion provided a handy excuse for the timing of an already scheduled, unselective armed attack.

The failure of the inmates to execute the hostages, an act they were in position to carry out in the first minutes of the assault, when it was clear that they themselves faced certain

death, falsified the argument that this was the only way to save
the hostages' lives. The belief that a hard line would keep the
state's authority from being undermined proved wrong: there
was a marked proliferation of prison rebellions across the country in the wake of the recapture of Attica. The decision to go
in was based on badly thought out reasons; but it was not a
frivolous decision, and that makes the action all the more sinister. The best that can be said is that the authorities were unaware that the hostages were still alive.

I could have gone to Attica to see firsthand what had happened. I couldn't quite pin down a reason for the hostility with
which Dr. Edland's report had initially been greeted and thought
I might get some insight if I could talk to people firsthand. But
I accidentally overheard a conversation between my two sons
that made me realize that I didn't belong at Attica. "Has Dad
been on any ego trips lately?" one asked the other. I took a
long, hard look at myself. Was I taking assignments just to be
part of the action? Attica was a deadly serious business, and
it would have been irresponsible for me to go unless I was really
needed.

So, when I was asked on three different occasions to come
to Attica, after careful thought I refused. There were competent
pathologists already there; my presence would simply have
added to the confusion.

A wild combination of wind and rain started a chain of
thought that led me to the heart of the Attica matter. I had
finished the day's work at Brookdale Hospital and was driving
home in the midst of a sudden storm. By the time I crossed
the Manhattan Bridge, traffic was at a standstill. Later I learned
that traffic was completely snarled both in and around the city.
It took four hours for a twenty-five-minute trip. I was stuck
alone in the car; it was impossible to pull over to the side and
park. All I could do was wait, move the car a few feet every

so often, and sit and think. The hundreds of drivers going no-where, with the motors running, uselessly consuming fuel and polluting the air, prompted me to review my personal exposure to waste that day. It had begun at breakfast in the hospital cafe-teria. By the time I'd finished eating, my tray was cluttered with disposable plastic plates, knife, fork, spoon, orange-juice con-tainer, and cottage-cheese container, opened packets of salt, pepper, and sugar, a disposable coffee cup, and two paper napkins. These were dumped into a disposable plastic bag lining the vast cavity in the garbage compressor.

When I went to my office, my desk was covered with yester-day's junk mail: six drug-house-sponsored magazines, five pamphlets advertising the latest cures, five solicitations from "charitable" organizations, two bills from medical societies, five announcements of various meetings, six memos from several minor administrators, and a thick catalogue from an electronics-equipment manufacturer. To this I added the morning news-paper, and the wastebasket was completely stuffed.

Next I went into the tissue-cutting room, where five young doctors, members of my house staff, and two associates were waiting to review the morning's surgical specimens, just brought in from the operating rooms. We all put on disposable latex gloves, after taking each pair out of individual double wrap-pings. A disposable knife blade was removed from an aluminum-foil container and placed on the knife handle. The cut pieces of tissue were placed in individual plastic disposable cages (one hundred of these were used that morning) and dropped into a large bucket filled with formalin poured from a disposable gallon-size bottle. The session over, we threw our gloves, which had been used once, into a plastic bag lining the trash can. This routine was to be repeated several times that day.

When a call came for a consultation from one of the surgeons, I put on an operating-room gown before entering the operating room, a disposable mask, a disposable cap, and disposable shoe covers. In the OR the patient was draped with disposable sheets and towels. Blood in a disposable plastic bag was flowing into the patient's arm veins via a disposable tube and needle. The anesthetist was injecting medication from a disposable vial into the patient's other arm with a disposable syringe and needle. The anesthetic gas passed from a cylinder through disposable piping and into the patient's mouth through a disposable mask. The consultation finished, I left the OR and discarded the disposable items into a huge trash basket lined with a disposable plastic bag.

Back again in the office, I dictated my findings and had five Xeroxed copies made. They would be read once, folded, and then thrown away. I made a few notes with a disposable ballpoint pen.

Time for lunch. At the end of lunch I again emptied the tray with all its disposables; this time there was a disposable soda can added to the usual collection of waste.

The afternoon's activities were a repeat of the morning's, with the addition of an autopsy. The body was brought into the dissecting room clothed in a disposable paper shroud that was torn off and discarded. At the post-mortem examination, again we used disposable gloves, knife blades, containers, and aprons. Only a few years ago, durable rubber gloves and aprons were used; they were repeatedly washed and reused, and lasted many months. The knives were resharpened and served us for several years. Now everything is disposable. At the end of the dissection a new disposable paper shroud was placed on the body.

While I had been thinking all this in stop-and-go traffic, I had driven a few blocks, to Houston Street, where again I was blocked by a chaotic, intertangled mess of cars, trucks, and buses at the intersection. Now my stream of thought turned back to the mid-fifties, when our government stored tons and tons of "surplus" butter in caves, dumped vast mountains of bumper-crop wheat into the ocean, plowed under acre upon acre of ripe produce, and bribed farmers to make barren thousands of fields of fertile soil.

I thought of how these useless things and this waste make for useless and wasted people. And this led directly into my next mental exercise, concerning those members of the human "race" whom we routinely dispose of by removing them from the mainstream of our lives and from compassionate human care: the elderly, your parents and mine, exiled to dismal institutions for the aged and unkempt nursing facilities; the deformed or retarded placed in cold storage in human warehouses like Willowbrook; the prisoners isolated in a dehumanized and antiquated jailhouse system; the mentally disturbed discarded into the snake pits deliberately placed in inaccessible, outlying areas; and the minority peoples confined in hopelessness and despair to the rotting urban ghettos strung across the nation.

And then my thoughts returned to Attica, and suddenly it all fell neatly and horrendously into place. It was now clear why Attica was different, why the anguish is not yet extinguished and why people still refuse to believe the facts of the event. Attica makes a qualitative leap in our throwaway society. At Attica it was not the freaks, the outcasts, the criminals, who became expendible, for they always have been; but it was the "middle Americans," the "silent majority," the backbone of the country—the prison guards—who had entered the list of disposables. This was the singular ingredient that set the whole thing into proper and logical perspective. That is why the families of the dead hostages and society as a whole refused to accept as true Dr. Edland's findings that the guards, their own husbands, brothers, or sons, the men on the right side of law and order, had been disposed of by their own duly elected leaders.

Lest this evaluation of the Attica affair and its ultimate meaning seem an illogical, wild intellectual gyration, I offer in evidence the brilliant and insightful analysis that appeared in the

form of a New York *Times'* book review of three books on
Attica: *Attica—My Story,* by Commissioner Russell Oswald; *Attica—The Official Report of the New York State Commission
on Attica,* chaired by Robert McKay, Dean of New York University Law School; and *A Bill of No Rights—Attica and the
American Prison System,* by Herman Badillo and Milton
Haynes. Bryce Nelson, a Los Angeles *Times* correspondent and
the review's author says: "The inmates made a foolish misjudg-
ment of character when they thought that Governor Rockefeller
and his subordinates cared more about correctional officers than
they did about exterminating a supposed challenge to the political order. Behind the prison walls, as in Vietnam, our political
leaders are determined to preserve the state's reputation for
toughness without worrying much about human lives."

For one brief moment the outcasts, the hardened criminals,
and the anti-social psychopaths, by not instantly slashing their
hostages' throats, revealed more humanity than those who made
the decision to go in.

Bertrand Russell once said: "How comes it that human beings, whose contacts with the world are brief, personal and limited, are nevertheless able to know as much as they do?" And
the next logical question, to me, is: How comes it that human
beings, exposed to the vast accumulated experience and wis-
dom of man's lengthy sojourn on earth and also to the impact
of the trials and tribulations in their own personal lives, are
nevertheless unable to profit from these and keep on making
the same mistakes over and over again?

I hope we can learn to stop making mistakes before we make
so many that people stop caring altogether. It would be horrible
to succumb to the depressing view of history that says: "History always repeats itself, the first time as tragedy, the second
as farce."

INDEX